A TalkManTalk Book

FREE YOURSELF FROM YOURSELF

FAIL-PROOF PRINCIPLES FOR ADDICTION RECOVERY

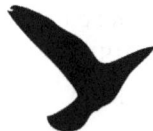

TIMOTHY STEWART

"The Addiction Rehab Coach"

First Hardcover Edition 2020
First Paperback Edition 2020
First Digital Edition 2020
TalkManTalk Publishing

Interior Design by Robert Smyth
Cover Design by Carol Phillips

For information regarding special discounts for bulk purchases, please contact TalkManTalk Publishing at info@talkmantalk.com. For more information about the author, visit freeyourselffromyourself.com.

Library of Congress Cataloguing in Publication Data

Stewart, Timothy.
  Free Yourself From Yourself: Fail-proof Principles for Addiction
  Recovery
  1. Nonfiction—Self-help—Health
  2. Addiction Recovery
I. FREE YOURSELF FROM YOURSELF
LC 2020915028

HARDCOVER ISBN: 978-1-7354829-0-3
PAPERBACK ISBN: 978-1-7354829-1-0
E-BOOK ISBN: 978-1-7354829-2-7

For Nana,
Evangelist Cleo Stewart

TABLE OF CONTENTS

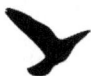

CONTENTS CONTINUED

FOREWORD

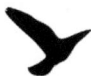

I have known Timothy Stewart for more than fifteen years. In addition to building our website and being our director of communications, he has taught Bible class and helped our community in numerous ways. In the time I've been his pastor, I've always known Timothy to work tirelessly to encourage others to have a positive outlook—especially when working with addicts and their families. He's helped numerous members of our congregation to understand addiction by bringing a powerful message of freedom from addiction and hope through the understanding and application of spiritual principles.

This understanding and application of spiritual principles is the foundation of Timothy's work as an addiction sponsor/coach, and it is an important part of recovery. Since the beginning of time, mankind has experienced ups and downs in all seasons of life. There are two ways people navigate their way through these peaks and valleys: with positive thinking or with negative thinking.

Negative thinking and constant self-criticism can destroy one's true self, conceal one's inner gift, and/or hinder one's productiveness in life. Self-induced destructive behaviors and unproductive perspectives can destroy one's future. Conversely, positive, healthy thinking is key to securing a good, solid sense of character and builds a solid foundation for achieving greater things. But true success starts within the heart.

We all have something precious, powerful, and purposeful inside us. It is not God's intent for that gift to remain hidden, unknown, and untapped. The book of Proverbs discusses "guarding our hearts." The writing suggests that life and personal development starts from the heart.

How we think, perceive, and process information from our many experiences informs how we see ourselves and how we can believe in ourselves. Becoming educated about healthy mental practices enables us to free ourselves from debilitating behaviors, unfruitful mindsets, and negative thinking. In freeing ourselves from those "mental handcuffs" or "invisible mind shackles," we learn how to detach from toxic thinking and, as a result, from toxic living.

Freedom from a lifestyle of active addiction begins with taking in the right new information that yields behavior modification, a direct result of our moral character. In this book, Timothy Stewart, an experienced sponsor/life coach in the addiction and recovery process shares his personal experiences and provides knowledge, insights, and practical tools to help liberate readers from negative addictive behaviors. Timothy presents a workable program devoted to character development, a process that helps people change the way they think. Remember: we are what we think.

—Dr. J. Sims, Ed.D., CEO, consultant, pastor

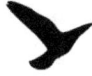

ACKNOWLEDGEMENTS

Writing *Free Yourself From Yourself* has been an incredible journey. Though it was birthed from my hard-won life experiences, many people helped me on the pathway toward recovery and later, success, and I'd be remiss if I didn't thank them for their support.

First, I'd like to thank Allen B. for sponsoring me over the course of many years. Sponsorship is the backbone of any recovery plan, and your wisdom and advice was invaluable to me. Thank you for guiding me through the steps over and over again, being an example for me in regards to how to live clean and sober no matter the circumstances, and becoming one of my best friends. My love and respect is yours.

Second, thank you to Chris R. & Harvey C., two of my closest comrades, for all we've shared on and off the field of recovery. I love and respect you guys with all that I am. We will be the three amigos for life!

Third, my mentors—Gary R. Blair, Ron Stokes, Dr. Julius R. Sims, and Rev. Phil Brickle—thank you for all of the time you have invested in my development over the years and all of the wisdom you have continued to pour into my soul. This book would not have become a reality without your support. I am so very grateful to each of you for your continued love, encouragement, and direction.

Fourth, I'd like to extend a special thank you to my St. Louis recovery family members in the NA, CA, and AA. Unfortunately, there are too many names to list here, but I am so grateful for each and every one of you. When I had no one, you were there for me and certainly helped save my life. I will always be grateful for you.

Fifth, Jevon R., thank you for all of our late-night conversations and for sharing many of life's joys and pains with me these past seven years. You have been an inspiration and a true-blue friend; I have never shared so much laughter with anyone else on this planet. Your honesty and friendship has helped me remain free from denial.

Sixth, I would also like to acknowledge Danielle Featherson for helping me craft my rough draft and for putting up with hours and hours of interviews and conversations. Thank you to my beta readers, for listening to my story, reading multiple drafts of this book, and providing valuable feedback. And finally, thank you to Jessica and her editorial team at Brigid Book Works for helping me bring this book to fruition. Your team is amazing!

Lastly, I'd like to acknowledge my parents, daughters (Raven and Danielle), and family members who have motivated me in one way or another to never give up. And to my future readers, thank you for reading this book. I hope the Free Yourself From Yourself program inspires you to make lasting positive changes in your lives. I'm rooting for you!

INTRODUCTION

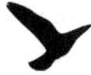

I lived trapped in active addiction for more than twenty-five years of my life. For much of that time, I didn't realize I was caught up in the grip of what I now know as "active addiction." For many years, I was a functional addict; however, addiction is so cunning, baffling, and powerful, for a long time I didn't even know I had crossed that invisible line from recreational using into full-blown addiction.

I started smoking marijuana at the tender age of twelve. I had been warned by my great-grandmother that if I continued smoking marijuana, before long I would be using that "hard stuff," as she called it. She was right! Over the years, those "little" joints I regarded as just something I smoked to get high with progressed, leading to drinking alcohol and then onto using cocaine. Eventually, I even graduated to smoking crack cocaine.

I was a pretty intelligent kid and adolescent. From a young boy to a teenager to a young adult, I always made good grades, and was even on the honor roll several times. I was an all-county trumpet player in the school band, and I earned a high test score on the ASVAB that allowed me to join the US Air Force. Years later, I got married, had a daughter, and lived a somewhat functional existence. Until I didn't.

Eventually, life became a living hell for me. I reached a point where I honestly didn't care whether I lived or died, and I didn't feel anyone else cared either, except for my nana and my granddaddy John. On many days, I cried out loud, "God, why did you let this happen to me again? Why?" I blamed God and anyone else I could for all the hell and misery in my life, but the reality was that neither God nor anyone else was to blame for me continuing in this condition. I was the culprit. This was my doing, but I didn't know how to face this reality, and I didn't have the courage to accept responsibility for this lifestyle nor the results from it.

During my twelfth (yes, *twelfth*) rehab, I came to the harsh realization that I didn't know how to live. I could exist. I could survive. But I didn't know how to live. This realization was heartbreaking and left me feeling dumbfounded and numb. But I knew I had to make a decision to either learn a new way to live or to die in the horrors of active addiction.

Instead of blaming everyone around me, I started to look at the real cause. What I realized was that there was a "root cause" behind why I was using and abusing drugs, alcohol, and people. The substances weren't the issue. The issue was my way of thinking and the habits this thinking created, which controlled my behavior. Only when I began to absorb new, healthy information, change my thinking patterns, and create new habits that produced different behaviors and results, was I able to free myself from myself and become the responsible, productive member of society that I am today.

As humans, how we think is determined by our environment and the information our environment subjects us to, which we continue take in again and again, and over time the environment we've surrounded ourselves with creates our philosophy and ultimately our habits. Research proves that 80 percent of our decisions are based on how we feel, which dictates our actions. We are creatures of habit, although not all habits are bad habits. Our thoughts create and develop our habits, and our habits define our future. We don't decide our future; we decide our habits. And our habits dictate our future.

I grew up on a 500-acre farm, and I've discovered that human functionality operates very similar to the process of sowing and reaping. Words and deeds are to our soul like seeds are to soil: If we plant an apple seed and it sprouts, we're going to get an apple tree. If we plant a pumpkin seed and it sprouts, we're going to get a pumpkin plant. If, throughout our lives, our environment—the people and events around us—sows seeds of negativity, immorality, and depravity, that's the kind of harvest that's going to be produced in our lives, which will lead to unethical and unhealthy behaviors. Changing those negative behaviors at the seed level and producing healthy thought patterns that create productive habits and behaviors is what *Free Yourself From Yourself* is all about.

In this book, I share my experiences with addiction and act as your personal coach to help you through your own addictions. Through exercises, I encourage you to take a look at those early seeds that were planted within you and that continued to be planted every day. After we root out the bad seeds, or "weed" seeds, if you will, I help you to begin planting healthy seeds that lead to moral thinking, healthier habits, and respectable behaviors. My goal is to help guide you to a more positive path and to ultimately living the life you were meant to live from the day you were born.

In the first part of this book, I relate my personal battles with active addiction and how it all started for me. In the second part, I outline how I freed myself from active addiction and continue to do so on a daily basis—because we live free from the grip and control of our addiction one day at a time. Here, I use anecdotes from my own experiences to illustrate the spiritual principles I discovered that can help you on your recovery journey. These principles are the foundation of the 12-step program, the basis for the majority of recovery programs in our society today. While learning and practicing the principles in these steps, I've gained knowledge for how to live my life. As of the writing of this book, I have been living clean and sober for sixteen years. By sharing my story with others, I have been able to help many find their way to recovery. My goal is to help you get to a place where you can live your life the way you want, free from the horrors of active addiction.

After I explain each spiritual principle in detail, I also include a practical exercise to help you apply the knowledge you've learned and take action. These exercises are designed to help you through the recovery process. Most of these exercises involve writing, so keep a notebook or a journal handy as you work your way through this program. Some of the exercises you will want to revisit again and again because, as I said, sobriety is a lifelong commitment.

In this book, which is the starter guide to my Free Yourself From Yourself Program, I will explain how understanding and applying these 12 core spiritual principles in my daily life worked for me, as they will for anyone, and deliver coaching tips to help get you or a loved one started on the road to recovery.

Addiction programs talk a lot about a Higher Power. Some choose to think of this Higher Power as "This Big Guy in the Sky," otherwise known as God. This Higher Power for you does not have to be that particular "God." What I suggest is choosing a Power that will help you look beyond yourself, a loving and caring Power that gives you a good, positive direction for your life.

When I started recovery, the Christian God was my Higher Power. As I learned more about the spiritual principles in the 12-step program, which are derived from the Bible, and more about myself, my Higher Power evolved into something different. But I still use God as an acronym to represent this power:

Good

Orderly

Direction

For me, having a Higher Power means having a deep understanding of and living the spiritual principles that give me my Good Orderly Direction. Living this way helps me make decisions that keep me from causing myself and others pain that requires medication. While they're derived from the Bible, and while I do reference biblical scriptures throughout the book, the principles are more like a map that anyone who is willing to change can follow.

"What is a spiritual principle?" you ask. I'm glad you asked. It took me a bit of time to come up with an understanding of these principles before I could incorporate them in my life. Let's take a look at the dictionary to see if it can lend us some clarity and understanding. The *Oxford Handbook of Psychology and Spirituality* provides two relevant definitions. First, *spiritual* is defined as "relating to, consisting of, or affecting the animating or vital principle held to give life to physical organisms." In layman's terms, the *spiritual* is something that gives life, or affects the will to live. Second, *principle* is defined as "a comprehensive and fundamental law, doctrine, or assumption." So, putting these two together, I constructed a simple, solid, working definition of a spiritual principle for us to use: *spiritual principles* are fundamental laws that guide our decision-making process, helping us live a lifestyle of morality and integrity, thereby defining our purpose and will to live.

Make no mistake. Even though I have been clean and sober for more than sixteen years, my goal remains progress rather than perfection. Breaking free from active addiction is always a work in progress, but it is achievable and sustainable. I did it, and you can too. This book is designed to help you or someone you love struggling with addiction get started on the path toward recovery. By following these spiritual principles, using my program, and engaging in personal coaching, you can discover, create, and nurture the habits that will deliver a brighter future and a better life.

PART I

MY ADDICTION

PART I: MY ADDICTION

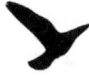

What makes me qualified to help guide others on the road to freeing themselves from their addiction or addictions? It's because I've done it. I've lived it. I've suffered it. And I've overcome it, one day at a time. I'm not speaking from a podium like an academic with a string of degrees. I lived through some tough times and terrible situations. I've made some bad mistakes, but by getting on the path of recovery, I learned some principles to live by, and when I followed those principles, I was able to come out on the other side. Since then, I've helped many others free themselves from active addiction. If I can do it, and they can do it, I firmly believe you can too.

In recovery programs such as Narcotics Anonymous (NA), Alcoholics Anonymous (AA), and Free Yourself From Yourself (FYFY), we use a common language and common terms to aid with our discussions. Here are some definitions to important words that we need to fully understand as we work through the information provided in this book:

- *Addiction*: a sick psychological and pathological reaction to anything with life-damaging consequences, not limited to drugs and alcohol.
- *Obsession*: a fixed idea or emotion that predicts, dictates, or controls one's life and behavior.
- *Compulsion*: the inability to stop once started.
- *Denial*: refusing to admit the truth or reality of something unpleasant.

You'll hear these words a lot throughout our discussion, so try to commit their meanings to memory. In this section, I'll share with you some of my story. In the next section, I'll share more details that help support the spiritual principles I've learned in my recovery to help free anyone from the horrors of active addiction.

So, why am I known as "the addiction rehab coach?" Because with this book and my Free Yourself From Yourself program, I will be on the sidelines sharing, coaching, guiding, and cheering you on every step of the way. I can do this because I know exactly what addiction feels like, and I know what it takes to get to the pathway of recovery. You will get there.

CHAPTER ONE: WHERE IT STARTED

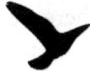

I'm originally from North Carolina. I grew up on a 500-acre farm where we grew corn, soybeans, wheat, peanuts, watermelon, and a variety of vegetables. We had nine turkey houses and a hog house. I didn't just grow up there, though. I worked on the farm and that farm worked on me. It shaped me into a unique young man.

I had a lot of responsibility as a young person because my grandfather owned the farm. I had to get rid of dead turkeys and wash out the turkey waters every day after school, a nasty, dirty job that took hours. I also had to cut grass, split wood, disk land, and on top of that, sometimes I had to make sure the other guys were doing their work.

My life as a kid was a little unusual because when other kids got home from school they played, watched TV, rested, or did their homework, but when I got home, I had to go to work. I had visited the homes of two of my best friends, Ricky and Avery, on several occasions, and I saw that their families operated very differently. However, in our family culture, I had no choice but to work. We did what we were told to do. At the end of the day, when we were eating dinner, I wasn't asked, "How did you do in school today?" Instead, the question was, "Did you get all of your work done?"

As the firstborn and first grandchild to my grandparents on both sides, expectations for me were pretty high. My grandfather introduced me to the great outdoors. He taught me how to hunt and fish, how to drive tractors, and how to value hard work. He entrusted me with a lot of responsibility from a very young age. Oftentimes, it was up to me to ensure that our hired hands got their work done. On many occasions, he told me what he wanted other farmhands to do, and I had to make sure they did it.

My grandfather had only a sixth-grade education, but he achieved quite a bit for himself and our family. In addition to having this farm, we had a general store. The store was located in a long green building in the fork of two roads, where my grandfather also lived, and we used that building to generate a few other revenue streams. We ran a general store with a kitchenette in the back where we sold cooked food, beer, and hard liquor, which was illegal. Down the hall from the kitchenette, we ran a disco club where people from our town and surrounding towns would come on the weekends at night to let loose—people I knew, like teachers, other farmers, businessmen, and even clergymen. Then, behind the disco club was our motel, where couples headed after leaving the club.

As a kid I hung out with customers from our store, other farmers, and the full-time guys who worked on the farm. They were all middle-aged men. As you might imagine, I was exposed to quite a bit while still at a young, tender age.

On weekends, when people came to the club, I had the chance to see what a lot of the older folks did at night, away from their normal lives. Even people who were well-respected in our community lived a different lifestyle at our club. They let their hair down, drinking and smoking and dancing, and sometimes they even headed to the motel afterward with people other than their spouses.

Because this dysfunction was going on where I lived, and all around me, I was introduced to immorality in a visceral way. I saw some things firsthand that kids my age didn't know anything about. When I was twelve, because my playmates were forty- and fifty-year-old farmhands who ended the day smoking and drinking, I grew up very quickly. So quickly that when I was sixteen, my mom told me that I already had the mindset of a thirty-year-old. I was so much more advanced than my peers, in so many ways, and in many ways which were not good, as I found out years later.

I started smoking cigarettes at age eleven. Everyone I knew—my grandfather, father, mother, the farmhands, and the clubbers I hung out with—smoked cigarettes, so it seemed normal for me to smoke. Of course, they told me not to smoke, but that didn't matter. If they could smoke, I reasoned that so could I. I just couldn't get caught. I wasn't doing what I was told, but I was doing *what I was shown.*

In school, I was constantly in trouble. I was naturally inquisitive and mischievous. I think I had ADHD, but no one knew what that was back then. I didn't know why I did the things I did, but despite being in trouble all the time, I did well in school. I got As or Bs, even though I rarely studied. I didn't make the time to study because I had to work all the time, and as I already explained, no one in my family seemed to care about my grades that much anyway. School wasn't that important. They taught me what they knew. Remember that my grandfather hadn't gone to school past the sixth grade and my parents had only graduated from high school. According to my family, a man who worked hard could have anything he wanted, and that was what they preached and taught me daily.

They didn't really support any of my academic or creative endeavors because they simply didn't think they were necessary. I can remember my first two instances of real emotional pain as a kid. They were the greatest disappointments of my childhood and adolescence. How I processed the emotions from these events would frame my thinking and my way of coping with pain and loss for many years to come.

My first story begins in Ms. Jenkins's fifth-grade classroom. Five students had been selected to work on a special art project that was going to the White House to be presented to the president. And I was one of those students. This project was a big deal, not only for our class, but also for the school. All five of us were relocated to our own special section at the front of our classroom, where we would work on the project together. We were instructed that we would have to stay after school in order to complete the project in the allotted time. I was so excited because Ms. Jenkins had recognized that I was a gifted little boy.

When I got home from school that day, I changed into my work clothes, ran down to where my dad was, all out of breath, to tell him the good news. When I told him I had to stay after school and would need him to pick me up, he looked at me and said, "You know I can't come out to that school in the afternoon to pick you up, I have to work." Immediately, for some reason, I felt a hurt that I had never experienced before, and all of my excitement vanished instantly. I could not believe he was saying these words to me. I knew I would not be able to work on the project because Ms. Jenkins had made it very clear that we would have to stay after school and be picked up by our parents.

The next morning on the school bus, I was still very hurt because I would have to tell Ms. Jenkins I could not stay after school and now I would be embarrassed in front of the entire class. One of the other students selected, Diane, happened to ride my bus. Evidently she saw the hurt on my face, and she asked me what happened. When I told her I didn't have a ride home, she said, "Don't worry. My mom will bring you home. You can ride with us." My excitement reengaged instantly; I could now stay on the project and my dad did not have to come pick me up. I had a ride home. When I arrived at school, I explained to Ms. Jenkins what my dad said, but I also explained that I could still work on the project because I could ride home with Diane. So she allowed me to continue to work with our group that day.

When I got home that afternoon, I changed into my work clothes, ran down to tell my dad the good news, all excited again, and my dad looked at me and said, "Who's gonna wash out these turkey waters? You can't stay after school. You've gotta come home and wash out these waters." I was speechless! This time, the hurt went even deeper because I knew this was the real reason my father wouldn't let me work on the art project in the first place: he needed me to come home and go to work. At first I was kind of numb, then I became angry. I went and hid and smoked some cigarettes. I'd seen my uncles and some farmhands smoking weed, and I started thinking about where I could find some.

The next day, I had to tell Ms. Jenkins that I could not stay after school. She said she understood, but she would have to choose another student to work on the project. So I had to move all of my things back to the regular class section, and I was very embarrassed. I think the entire classroom felt my pain. Everyone was super quiet as I packed my things.

A few days later, I did find a weed connection with some older guys who came to our store, and I became a regular customer who smoked weed daily. I was twelve years old, and I was already using a substance to cope with my disappointment. Soon I had used up my allowance, and

I started stealing money when I needed to in order to keep an ongoing supply of weed.

At this point, I became a bad boy. I became a deviant, a thief, and a sneak, and I didn't care. Every time something didn't go my way, I got high. It helped me forget the so-called unfairness of my situation. I began to fight often on the bus and at school, making a name for myself as the cool guy who kept money, smoked weed, and liked to fight. "That's cool-ass Tim Stewart," they would say, and I was way okay being that kid.

I did get caught, of course, several times. My parents would find my stash, and my father would beat me and send me out to do more work. But that didn't stop me. I'd just acquire more weed and smoke away the pain again as soon as I got the chance.

The second biggest disappointment of my youth happened when I was a teenager. One day, after I beat up another student right in front of the principal at my junior high school, my dad received a call. Mr. Henry, who was one of my dad's teachers when he was in school, but was now the principal. My dad came down to the schoolhouse to pick me up and Mr. Henry told my dad he had never seen a kid attack another kid with such ferocity, I could just see the disappointment and embarrassment on my dad's face. I had already been expelled from school three times for fighting in the past two years, so he suggested that I join an extracurricular activity and apply some of my energy toward something good.

I guess my dad heard Mr. Henry's suggestion, and he got me into the band that summer. My dad wanted me to play the sax, but I wanted to play the trumpet because he had played the trumpet when he was in school. I knew I got into a lot of trouble, but for some reason, I still wanted my parents to be proud of me.

So I began taking trumpet lessons, and my skills developed quickly. My band director, Mr. Taylor, was so impressed that he added me to the high school marching band while I was still in junior high school. During our half-time show at our home football games, I often performed a solo. I was a darn good trumpet player, and I loved it. Even though I was still getting high every day, playing my trumpet had become another outlet for me, a release from the hard work associated with farm life.

Every year, all of the school bands from each town in our county would meet to audition for "chairs" in the All-County band for a one-night concert. I believe the concert was a fund-raiser for our school district. At any rate, many important people attended and everyone was dressed to impress. I made all-county band for three years in a row, and by my second year I had won first chair out of over 200 trumpet players.

In my sophomore year, Mr. Taylor said that he was positive he could help me get a scholarship at Campbell University through the band, because he knew the band director there personally, but he said I needed to upgrade my trumpet to better my skill and tone. He showed me a Bach Stradivarius trumpet, and it was gorgeous. The shiny silver instrument would certainly help me stand out among the other trumpet players, but it cost $300.00.

I went home and told my parents what Mr. Taylor had said. They replied they did not have the money. So I went to ask my grandfather. Remember, my grandfather owned a lot of land and had many different streams of revenue. He was known for having money to help other people. I even arranged for Mr. Taylor to speak with my grandfather over the phone when I went to ask him for the money. When he got off the phone, he said, "I don't have the money to buy no trumpet for you."

I just looked at him.

This was the same hurt I had felt back in grade school when I was not able to work on the art project, but I was a big boy now. I didn't show how hurt I was. I didn't even ask why he'd refused. I just walked out of the store. I walked back across the street to our house, went upstairs, grabbed my trumpet, slung it in the attic, and never picked it up again. I quit the band. I knew my parents wouldn't care. Besides, now that I no longer had practice, I had more time to smoke weed.

Forty years later, I can still remember these events as if they happened yesterday. Of course, I can't totally blame my addiction and everything that went wrong in my life on these two incidents. I continued to make the *choice* to cope with my pain by abusing substances. At a very young age, I had already developed a very unhealthy way to handle disappointments and emotional pain . . . I got high. It became my tried-and-true coping mechanism.

I took college prep courses in high school because I had some great teachers who thought a lot of me and who thought I would do well academically on the collegiate level. They seemed to believe I had a lot of potential, but I don't think they really knew how to connect with me. Besides, I didn't want to go to college because I didn't want to have to come home during the summer and work on the farm. When I left home, I wanted to leave. I needed another plan.

My uncle David and my uncle Wiggy were probably my biggest heroes growing up, especially Uncle Dave. He had been a Marine, and he was exciting. He was in great shape. He was the family protector and he was a fighter. He lived in New York and, along with my aunt Pat, ran the store my family owned in Brooklyn, another one of my grandfather's businesses. I always wanted to be like my uncle Dave.

Uncle Wiggy, on the other hand, was the nice guy that everybody liked. He was a veteran of the US Navy, and he got along with anyone. He was the kind of man who could make everyone laugh and who would give the shirt off his back to someone in need, but if you ever crossed him, there would be hell to pay. Uncle Wiggy always took up for the underdog. He disliked anyone who mistreated others, and I certainly adopted that mindset, too. My personality became a product of these two guys—a real-life Dr. Jekyll and Mr. Hyde. I could be a real nice guy one minute, but I could rip your head off your shoulders the next minute if you crossed me or anyone I knew.

Throughout my childhood, I wasn't really close to my dad because I didn't want to be like him. He worked all day and night, the hardest-working man I have ever known. No one could outwork him. And he was okay with working on a farm and just being a regular kind of guy, but I was attracted to "flashy" things. He didn't want or need too much more; his work and his family were enough for him. My uncles, on the other hand, lived in New York and drove bright, shiny cars. Uncle Dave always had pretty women on his arm and lots of money in his pocket. I wanted that. I didn't want what I saw my dad doing. My uncles taught me many things about how to be a man, and maybe some things they shouldn't have taught me at such an early age. But they took time with me, didn't beat me, and when I was with them, I felt like I was hanging with the big boys!

Just like my uncles, I decided to join the military after high school. I took the ASVAB test and scored high enough to get into the Air Force. My family was more excited about this achievement than I was. They were probably tired of dealing with me. I was just happy I was getting away from that farm.

Once I was in the military, I was no longer connected to that dysfunctional environment. I began to experience life on an entirely different level. I went overseas. I spent two years in Europe, and this farm boy visited several countries where people spoke different languages and had entirely different cultures. It was an eye-opening experience, and I loved it.

In the Air Force, I was a medic first and then became an EMT. I was stationed in Germany, at Wiesbaden Regional Medical Center, and I was part of the Medevac team that brought marines who got bombed in Beirut back into Germany.

I traveled a lot of places while I was in the Air Force, including Russia, England, and France. I was in Germany before the wall came down in Russia, and life on the other side of that wall was bizarre and extraordinary, a far cry from my life on the farm.

Many of the younger guys I was stationed with would drink every day, but at the time, drinking really wasn't my thing. After all, I had been drinking since I was ten or eleven years old. Drinking wasn't new to me like it was to them. I never smoked pot or did any drugs while in the air force, though. My superior officers conducted random drug screenings all the time, and I wasn't about to risk getting kicked out of the military on a dishonorable discharge. I had at least some sense back then, and I have always had a lot of pride and ego.

When my military service was complete, I came back home. My intention was to marry my high school sweetheart, but that didn't work out. She had gotten pregnant and then had an abortion without even telling me until it was done. This experience caused me real emotional pain. And, to cope with it, I turned back to my old habits and the dysfunctional mindset that created a destructive lifestyle. I started hanging out with some folks who were into drugs, and I soon developed more new bad habits as my addiction progressed into full-blown addiction to hard alcohol and hard drugs.

Chapter Two: Where It Led

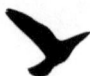

After the air force, I lived in several states and cities, and I was clean and sober at times, but the addiction always resurfaced because I didn't know how to live any other way. Though I didn't realize it, being an addict was as firmly rooted in me as anything I had been taught in my life, but I was in denial. It was a learned behavior that had now become a disease, and the only way I was going to be able to break this addiction was to change the behaviors that created it. But that wouldn't happen for almost twenty years. You can't fix something if you don't know how it works. For example, one thing a car mechanic must know in order to fix a car is how it's supposed to function under normal circumstances.

I didn't understand how to live my life in a healthy way. For a long time, I was what we call a "functioning addict." I still went to work and held down good jobs at world-class organizations like UPS and IBM. I got married, and even had a daughter. I would clean up for periods of time, but I always seemed to go back to my old ways. After my wife and I separated and then divorced, and I couldn't see my daughter, my whole world crashed in on me. I stopped being responsible. From that point, the drugs and alcohol took control over my life. I moved to live with my nana and granddaddy John in Newark, New Jersey, where drugs and alcohol were always right around the corner, day or night.

I was in such a bad way that my mom told me at one point, "Son, if you continue to live the life you're living, you're not going to make it. I want you to know that I bought a $10,000 insurance policy to bury you with 'cause you ain't gonna make it." She didn't believe I was going to survive, because I was running around on the streets of New York all day and all night, getting high, sometimes going without sleep for days. I think this was her way of preparing for the worst, but deep down inside,

I think she hoped her speech might be a wakeup call for me—and she was right. My dad didn't want to have anything to do with me, he was so embarrassed by my behavior. I didn't know how to stop doing what I was doing; I just didn't want to feel any pain. I thought that the drugs and alcohol were the problem. It took years before I understood that my thinking was the problem.

In those twenty or so years, living in the grips of active addiction, I can't tell you how many times I said, "I'm not going to do this anymore. I'm not going to do this anymore." Then I would quit for a little while, but I was deep in denial. I got into another relationship, and we had a daughter. Then, inevitably, I was lured back into the vicious cycle. That relationship ended as well, and more pain meant more alcohol and crack to numb the pain.

The only person who still believed in me during this time was my nana. I didn't even believe in myself any longer, and she was the only one who gave me some hope throughout these years. When the majority of my family members turned their backs on me and expressed their disappointment, my nana was always there with open, loving, and praying arms. She never turned her back on me or gave up on me, no matter what.

My nana was an Evangelist and very well respected among our family, friends, and community. She was often referred to as a "powerful woman of God." Whenever my life spiraled downward, I found myself at her doorstep, broken, beaten, and defeated. She always took me in, happy I was with her and not living on the streets, even though I still spent way too much time hanging out in the wrong places.

Nana prayed for me daily. There were many times I couldn't even look her in the eyes because of my shame and embarrassment, and I didn't want to see the hurt in her eyes because of my addictive behaviors and the hurt I'd caused her. She was not blind to the fact that I was an addict, but she believed in God, and she told me many times, over and over again, with tears in her eyes, "God's going to bring you out." I couldn't see a way out, and I didn't really know what she meant, but later I realized that she was patiently sowing a seed of faith and hope. I grew up in the church, but nana had this relationship with God like I had never seen before.

Eventually, I made a decision. I was working in Brooklyn at the family store, and I left work and called her from the bus station. I told her, "You know what, I need to do something different. I need to get away from everybody. I need to leave because I can't seem to stop using. I'm going to get some help."

One of the strongest motivating factors for this change was my daughters. I didn't want them growing up being told, "Your dad is a crack-head." That thought gave me enough motivation that I did not give up, even though I wanted to.

So, at the age of forty, I found myself at the end of the road. I prayed to God, "Let me just get away. Let me just try to get clean a different way."

I was feeling very lost, like I had to run away, as I did a lot in my active addiction years. But where to this time? I bought a one-way bus ticket to California, but I didn't make it that far. Instead, I ended up in St. Louis, Missouri. I had never been there, and I didn't know a soul.

The people in the NA program in St. Louis welcomed me with open arms, helping me accept the harsh reality that at age forty, I had lost everything because of my addiction. My family, my marriage, and my relationship with my children—all of these were gone. I was reduced to two pairs of pants, two shirts, and about eight dollars in my pocket when I landed at their doorstep. Years of active addiction had robbed me of everything I held dear, and I was mentally, physically, emotionally, and spiritually bankrupt. The denial was over, I was a addict! Life had become a living hell for me, and I honestly didn't care whether I lived or died at moments. I didn't feel anyone else really cared either.

There was a VA treatment facility in St. Louis, the John Cochran VA Medical Center, but because there was no room for me when I arrived, they sent me to the Salvation Army's homeless shelter to wait two weeks for an open spot in the program. The shelter had no beds available, so I had to sleep in the overflow area, on the floor, but it didn't matter too much. I was so numb from all the emotional pain and loss, I was an empty shell of a human being. Lying there many nights with tears running down my face, all I could think was, "Man, how in the world did I get here?"

This could not be all that life had to offer me. This could not be why I was placed on this earth—to feel this kind of pain. I knew plenty of people who led healthy lives, who had great careers, good marriages, and strong relationships with their families. But this just wasn't my story, and it hurt like hell.

I was ready to give up. I prayed, asking God, "Please take me out of here. I'm ready to go. I don't want to live anymore."

I was serious. That's how much pain I was in. It wasn't the only time I'd prayed for death. There were many times I'd tried to smoke enough crack for it to kill me. I wanted my heart to burst. From what I know about life now, and where I am mentally and emotionally, for a human being, any human being, to say, "I'm ready to die," because of pain and loss, that person is a very dangerous person to come into contact with.

Finally, I got a spot in what became my twelfth rehab program. This time, back in recovery, I rediscovered Narcotics Anonymous (NA) and the 12-step program. This time something happened, and a spiritual awakening sparked in me. I realized that all those years, I did not know *how* to live! I only knew how to survive; how to exist. But I did not know how to live. I realized that I had to make a decision to either learn a new way to live or die in the horrors of active addiction.

Sitting in the chow hall after dinner was served my first night at the VA Medical Center, I became angry thinking about my life. I sat up in the chair, and I hit my hand on the table. "God, why does this keep happening to me?"

At that moment, I heard a voice. It was as if God was speaking to me. Years later, I began to think of the voice as "my inner voice," but at that point, for me, it was the voice of God.

"Drugs and alcohol are not your problem," the voice said.

The voice did not say, "I got you. I love you. You're going to be okay." Instead, God just went straight to the point: "Drugs and alcohol are not your problem."

I sat up and I looked around. Even though I didn't audibly hear the voice, I felt like I did. I looked around. No one else was there.

"Okay. What's my problem then?" I asked.

"Your way of thinking is your problem," the voice replied.

Now I was really alert. I had gotten a direct response to my question. This voice, which came out of nowhere, had my full attention because I'd asked a direct question and received a direct response.

I don't know if you've ever been in a situation where you just felt like you were so alone, or in a situation where you needed some help and you didn't know where it was going to come from, and then all of a sudden a friend shows up and you think, "Thank God you're here." It was that kind of feeling, but ten times more powerful.

"Well, how should I think?" I asked.

"Think in line with my Word," the voice said.

At that, I got up and went back to my room, where I started looking for a Bible. I found one in the desk bedside the bed. I began to read and read down to Genesis 1:11: "And God said, 'Let every seed produce after its own kind.'"

The voice then spoke once more and said, "Words and deeds are just like seeds, they always produce after their own kind."

Now, that spoke to me. I was a country boy. I understood how planting seeds, caring for crops, and harvesting worked. Every time we sowed corn seed in the ground, we got corn. Every time we planted watermelon seeds, we got watermelons. I'd lived this tangible truth on the farm every season. Every seed produced after its own kind. Seed, time, and harvest. It would take years for me to fully understand that everything that grows is the result of a seed being sown. But the idea began to take root in my mind.

When the voice made that last statement, "Words and deeds are just like seeds, they always produce after their own kind," became a real turning point for me. This was the new operating system I would now live by. This was the foundational principle that would make my twelfth rehab a success:

Words and deeds are just like seeds, they always produce after their own kind.

This concept sparked the development of a brand-new philosophy and belief system for me. Now I began to understand that if I wanted right things to happen in my life, I had to do right things. I had to plant the right seeds—period!

The more I read the Bible, the more I understood where the principles of recovery, the basis of the 12-step program, came from. The value of the Bible, for me, came not in the stories it told, but in the lessons those stories delivered. These lessons are the spiritual principles we will start talking about in Part Two of this book.

Finally, I was on the pathway toward figuring out how to live and living a lifestyle based on spiritual principles. I was on my way to recovery.

Chapter Three: What I Learned

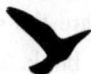

As I began the recovery process again, I looked back at my life and the decisions I had made. I realized I had landed in a lot of terrible situations because of my poor deeds, which produced poor results in my life. Some of the seeds that had been sown in me produced wrong thinking that created bad habits, and those bad habits produced ill behavior. My behavior was the reason I was living the lifestyle I lived. A person can say anything they want, but it's our behavior that tells the real story. Behavior never lies. The results of my behavior showed that I didn't know how to live. Survive, yes. But not live.

I began to realize that I was living off some of the bad information I had been given while growing up, and I had developed some unhealthy coping mechanisms in response. The people around me as I was growing up sometimes did things that were outside of the law and society's moral values. I grew up thinking it was okay to do a little wrong as long as I didn't get caught. Basically, I adopted that philosophy because that was the environment I was raised in and the ethical code that many lived by.

How deeply were those early lessons etched into my character and my thinking? If I got caught doing something wrong, I was beaten. So, I got punished, but all around me, I saw people do the things they told me were wrong. For example, I got beaten by my parents, who told me not to smoke, even though they smoked. What do you think that does to the mind of a young person? What kind of thought process does that create?

In recovery, while I revisited all of these memories, I started to understand that I was not responsible for the environment I was raised in and the lessons I was taught. But as a grown man, continuing to live out those lessons was purely on me. Sure, I had received some incorrect information in my younger years about how to live, but now I needed to know better so

I could do better. I needed to learn how to make better decisions. I needed to learn how to live my life based on truth and principles, not emotions.

I started to think about how I operated as a human being. What I came to learn is that I am a spirit, living in a body, and that I possess a soul. My soul is made up of my mind, will, and emotions. This was when I developed my concept of seed, time, and harvest, and when it became clear to me that my soul is just like soil. So, just like we planted corn and watermelon seeds in dirt, I was planting spoken words and daily deeds into my soul.

Just as the type of seed dictates what sprouts from the soil, the words and deeds sown into my soul dictate the choices I make and ultimately the results in my life. I know I can't be around people who use filthy language all day and not expect filthy language to come out of me. Instead, I need to be very careful of the seeds I allow to be sown into the soil of my soul. Planting good seed is only part of the process; proper maintenance of the soil—my soul—is essential to cultivating behaviors that produce positive results.

I learned that to free myself from myself, the right seeds had to be sown into the right type of soil, which meant I needed the right spiritual motives before I could plant the seeds of recovery. I had to work on the maintenance of my mind, will, and emotions, and that would become a lifelong process for me. We live in an environment where we're constantly receiving new information through our senses to our soul, and we have to be vigilant about filtering out the bad information and allowing in the good.

During my recovery, I stumbled upon the teachings of Dr. Myles Munroe. Dr. Myles had been a pastor for over thirty years and had authored more than sixty books. He was a father, a husband, and a world-renowned speaker on leadership development who mentored millions. Dr. Myles taught a message about how our hearts and souls are influenced by our environments. He explained that we have two minds, our conscious and our subconscious. Our subconscious mind is our true heart, which holds our values, records our truths and beliefs, and dictates how we act. Our senses are constantly providing information to our conscious mind, and if we aren't careful, all of this information then downloads into our subconscious minds, which is what controls human thought. He explained that we need to guard our hearts and our thoughts. That message really added to my understanding of my newfound philosophy, and how I could take control of my life. I needed to think the right thoughts.

That teaching truly resonated with me because it aligned with my understanding of seed, time, and harvest; of soul and soil. What we sow is what we reap. As Dr. Myles so aptly stated, "If we don't control what comes into our conscious mind, it will soon become a part of our subconscious mind, which is our heart and whatever gets 'programmed' there, is what will control a person whether they like it or not."

This means that if we plant bad words, we cannot get the right result. Bad seed equals a bad harvest. We are constantly exposed to different sights and sounds, information, and people, and we have to learn to focus on the information that will help us cultivate our soul's soil, yielding the best harvest from our seed, which is equivalent to good habits and behaviors.

Five years after I heard the voice and committed to living a lifestyle of sobriety and serenity based on spiritual principles, I was living in St. Louis with Alicia, a very attractive woman who became my best friend. Alicia believed in me from the first time we met, when I had nothing. When I looked in her eyes, I felt like there was nothing I couldn't accomplish, and she became a very significant piece of my recovery.

After getting married and living in an apartment for four years, we bought a very nice house in a retirement community. No one had lived in the house for two years, so the yard was kind of jacked up with weeds in the lawn.

I called a landscaper to come over and when he did, I told him proudly, "This is my house right here." I had a big smile on my face. I mean, this was my crib. In just these few short years, after going through a psychic change, I'd gone from homeless to homeowner. Of course I was proud. "But man, my yard is messed up," I told him. "Everybody else's yard looks immaculate because they're retired. They work on their yards all day, every day, and mine is standing out like a sore thumb."

"Yeah, Mr. Stewart. You definitely have a weed problem. Do you know the best way to get the weeds out of your yard?"

I replied, "Yeah, you spray 'em."

"No. That's one way to do it, but it's not the best way."

So I guessed again, "Pull 'em up?"

"That's another way you can do it, but it's not the best way."

"Man, you know, I grew up on a five-hundred-acre farm. I do know a little something about seed, time, and harvest. And I used to cut a lot of grass."

He said, "Yeah? Well, what's the best way to keep the weeds out of your lawn?"

I threw up my hands. "I don't know. Tell me."

The landscaper then said, "Mr. Stewart, the best way to keep the weeds out of your lawn is to sow the grass seeds so thick that the weeds can't take root." As soon as he told me that, I heard the voice again. That same voice I had heard five years before. The voice said, "This is what I told Joshua. Sow my word so that the weed seeds of fear, doubt, worry, and confusion can't take root."

Later I went to look up the passage the voice was referring to in my King James Bible. Joshua 1:8 reads, "This book of the law shall not depart out of thy mouth; but thou shalt *meditate* therein day and night, that thou mayest observe to do according to all that is written therein: for then thou shalt make thy way prosperous, and then thou shalt have good success."

The word *meditate* was translated from the Hebrew word *hagah*, which means to mutter the same thing over and over and over. As I speak these laws out loud, in meditation, these words, these spiritual seeds, go into my ears sowing the right seeds thick.

I was somewhat familiar with this scripture, as I had become a student of the Bible for the past five years. But on this day, that scripture connected to everything I had come to learn—everything that I had been believing and living. It was another moment of spiritual clarity. God, as I believed at the time, had spoken to me again, and I was exceedingly joyful about where I was in life in that very moment. I wanted to cry.

Before the landscaper left, he also explained that around the last two weeks of September and the first two weeks of October, homeowners aerate their yards and overseed. In other words, they sow seeds over seeds, sowing the grass seeds so thick that the weed seeds can't take root.

I understood sowing the grass seed thick in the springtime, but why would you want to sow grass seeds in October when the grass is getting ready to die? Here's why. When we sow the grass seed in October, it goes down into the ground, and during the winter months, the root system develops. It does not have to support the grass on top of the dirt. It can focus all its nutrients and energy on developing the root system, down there under the dirt. The grass looks brown. It's dead. But the root system under the ground is developing. By adding this extra seed down there, the grass roots become so thick, there's no room for any weeds. By March and April, the grass starts to turn green again and the root system is healthy and strong enough to support a healthy lawn.

Now think about this: When we have hard times in life, we're hurting. This pain can be the direct result of something we did or a situation beyond our control. Either way, it's up to us to make decisions on how to move on from there, and those decisions can extend the barren season or bring us out of it. If we don't have the right seeds sown thick enough to choke out the weeds, we'll extend that barren season.

For most of my life, that's what I did, I kept extending the barren season. The circumstances of my upbringing were beyond my control, but I extended my barren season well into adulthood by not choking out the weeds with the right seed. I wasn't living in freedom. I was living as a captive of despair, fear, doubt, worry, and confusion—weeds from weed seed.

In her bestselling book *Battlefield of the Mind*, Joyce Meyer explains that a normal mind isn't wandering and wondering, confused, doubtful and unbelieving, anxious and worried, judgmental, critical, or suspicious of others. She explains that a normal mind isn't passive either.

We don't let our minds just receive information as it comes along and do nothing all day. Nelson Mandela said that no one could ever lock up his mind. His captors locked up his body, but his mind was never locked up. We cultivate our thinking. I wasn't doing that, so the result was captivity to ill thinking that created bad habits that kept me trapped in active addiction.

When we sow seed, we don't see immediate crops. For days, we don't see anything, then all of a sudden, boom. The plant busts through the dirt.

Our job during that barren season is to build our root system, to establish our spiritual and moral infrastructure, and to develop our foundation so that when things do change—and change does always come, for either better or worse—we can support the new healthy change, whether that change be a new lawn, new opportunity, new job, new life partner, or newfound revenue stream.

I continually work to make my root structure thick. No weed seeds can take root. Even though some might get sown, they can't take root. We will always be exposed to weed seeds constantly, but we can certainly choke them out. With this foundation or formula for success, I can continue getting good results in my life, just by repeating the process of sowing healthy seeds and right deeds. The highest degree of freedom for me is not being controlled by people, situations, or circumstances. It's about me being in control of my life, me being able to make the right decisions, me managing my emotions and not allowing my emotions to manage me. Never are we less free than when our emotions rule us.

What I discovered on my journey to recovery is that the greatest form of self-abuse in this world comes from wrong thinking, bad habits, and ill behavior. Because I allowed weed seeds take root and become full-grown weeds, they strangled out the good things in my life. My broken marriages, broken family ties, and ruined career opportunities were all results of bad seeds and deeds. I was sleeping on the floor in a homeless shelter and repeatedly using a drug I didn't even like—all of these were results of my wrong choices and my wrong thinking, derived from bad seeds. That wrong thinking formed a prison that held me back from becoming a better man, a better husband, and a better father.

When I went to the other eleven centers for treatment, I thought the drugs and alcohol were the problem. It wasn't until the twelfth treatment that I understood they were only symptoms of the problem. By focusing only on the drugs and alcohol, I was going out into the yard of my life and cutting down the weeds at the surface level. The problem with that method, focusing on the drugs and alcohol, is that when we go back out to our yard a few days later, the weeds are back. I couldn't stay clean. The drugs and alcohol always came back into my life. I was not attacking the root of the problem, and the root problem was my thinking. The weeds came back because I didn't pull them up from the roots and I wasn't plant-ing enough good seed to choke out the new weed seeds.

I used to rob people. I used to hurt people. The more I hurt the people around me, the more pain I felt because I was causing them pain. Then I medicated that pain with crack; a lot of crack. And I was doing more hurtful things to get more crack, so that was causing me more pain. It was a vicious cycle. It's the same thing with any addiction—food, sex, gam-bling, spending—any kind of habit or activity that we engage in that is unhealthy for us as human beings and produces bad results.

If you're going through pain right now, I want to help you. I want to help you understand your situation and take steps to change it. If you're not in a painful place right now, I want to help you prepare for those moments in life when you may find yourself out of your element and caught off guard.

I am now better able to reach my goals in life, by practicing these principles I've learned and through teaching about how life works. The foundational principle is all about seed, time, and harvest, as I explained above. The second principle I need to share with you is that everything counts.

What do I mean by "everything counts"? I mean that every piece of gossip, every bit of music, every TV show I take in—it all matters. Every moment I spend around people who talk and act in ways that are contrary to the way I aspire to talk and act matters. Every errant thought I enter-tain on how to pay someone back for wounding my ego matters. Every careless word I let fall from my lips matters. All of these things count toward either helping me sow the healthy grass so thick that it chokes out the weeds of my life or toward feeding the weed seeds so that they grow deeper roots and take away from my life.

I can grow the kind of life that I want. If I want love, I just love on people. If I want money, then I become a person of value in the lives of others. If I want responsible employees, then I become a responsible employer.

When I was caught up in the grips of active addiction, *I didn't know how to live.* Once I was able to admit that I didn't know how life worked, I became determined to discover how it did. Today, here's how I live: if there's any part of my life that I am not comfortable airing on national television, then that's the area of my life I need to focus on changing.

Everything counts!

Are there things about your life you wouldn't want broadcast on national television? I'm not talking about things you might not share because they're private. I'm talking about those things you'd rather not share because the pain of their reality brings shame or regret.

Now you know about my trouble with addiction. Do you struggle with an addiction too? Have you been struggling to manage your life in any of these areas: finances, career, romantic relationships, relationships with family and friends, public contribution, personal development, physical environment, fun and recreation, spirituality, or health and fitness?

When we struggle to manage our lives, it's a sign that there may be some weeds popping up. We don't always recognize there's a problem until the weeds start to flourish and really stand out. But when we recognize those weeds, those poor results, we need to understand that they won't go away on their own. We have to nurture our lives so much that it chokes out the weeds. I can help you start to do that.

Our lives are a series of choices, and every day I have to choose to choke out those weed seeds so I don't eventually fall back into active addiction. There is no one-and-done solution for addiction recovery. This is a lifestyle that we live one day at a time for the rest of our lives.

So I want you to ask yourself: Am I ready to change my lifestyle? If you're ready, the next section will show you how.

PART II
YOUR RECOVERY

PART II: YOUR RECOVERY

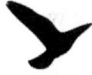

Bob Smith, MD, and Bill Wilson, an investor on Wall Street, were two very successful businessmen in their respective professions. Both were having issues with drinking. While they were both at a conference in Akron, Ohio, in 1935, they met each other in a bar. The conversation they shared changed the course of addiction treatment for good.

In their conversation, both men admitted that drinking had caused them problems and that they should not be drinking. They talked for a long time and before they knew it, it was three or four in the morning. The whole time they talked, they realized that neither of them had taken a drink.

They helped each other through that night, and afterward, they helped others. They put together a program based on principles from the Oxford Group movement, which was started by a Christian missionary and was very popular in the 1930s. Its founder was Christian, but the Oxford Group was a social group connected by a set of beliefs, not by organized religion.

Through understanding and application of the Oxford principles, Wilson and Smith formed the first Alcohol Anonymous groups. These groups proved for the first time in history that sobriety could be mass-produced, and they also prevented alcoholics from landing in institutions, which was how people with addiction issues had always been treated up to that time.

In this section, we will delve into the twelve principles that are at the foundation of any 12-step program, and I will show you how the understanding and the practice of these principles can help you in your recovery.

These principles worked for them, for me, and for millions of people who have freed themselves from all kinds of addictions and achieved clean and sober living through similar 12-step programs. The key is to fully understand the principles and spend each day applying them, because it is only through understanding and application that they work. I went through twelve rehab treatment programs before I understood that the 12 steps were not just about helping me step away from active addiction; they were about helping me change my way of *thinking*, so that I saw myself as someone trapped in active addiction.

When I finally understood how the 12 steps were about changing my thinking, and I applied this new way of thinking to every area of my life, not just those addictive urges, I was ready to fully understand and apply the universal principle of seed, time, and harvest.

You better believe I don't hang around crack houses today. That environment allows a toxic seeding into the soil of my soul, and I can't afford that kind of seed taking root in me. That toxicity is what we call weed seeds, and those weeds will strangle out the lush green lawn of positive habits and behaviors we work to grow within ourselves.

I don't need those kinds of weeds growing anywhere near my soil. Instead, I stay in environments that empower and challenge me to stay true to myself and my goals in life. Those are the kinds of seeds I want in the soil of my soul so that over time, I'll reap the kind of successful harvest I want.

So let's revisit our definition of *spiritual principles*. Remember, I combined two definitions to construct our own working definition:

- *Spiritual*: of, relating to, consisting of, or affecting the animating or vital principle held to give life to physical organisms.
- *Principle*: a comprehensive and fundamental law, doctrine, or assumption.

So, *spiritual principles* are fundamental laws that guide our decision-making process, helping us live a lifestyle of morality and integrity, thereby defining our purpose and will to live.

Spiritual principles are the fundamental laws we can live by. These principles covered in this section are the underlying messages of the 12 steps. Bob and Bill took principles found in the Bible and developed them into the steps of the 12-step program. Here we'll focus on the principles behind those steps, because they will give us a deeper understanding of what they mean, how to practice them, and how to apply them to our daily lives:

1. The Principle of Honesty
2. The Principle of Hope
3. The Principle of Faith
4. The Principle of Courage
5. The Principle of Integrity
6. The Principle of Willingness
7. The Principle of Humility
8. The Principle of Discipline and Action
9. The Principle of Forgiveness
10. The Principle of Acceptance
11. The Principle of Knowledge and Awareness
12. The Principle of Service and Gratitude

I've been practicing these principles for more than sixteen years, and I don't do them perfectly. No one does. But I do set my will each day to incorporate these principles in all of my affairs so I not only can stay free of my old toxic addictive thinking but also can set, achieve, and celebrate my new life goals.

This constant and vigilant application of spiritual principles is what helped me go from homeless to homeowner, what helped me begin to reconnect with my daughters after my addiction took me away from them, and what helped me go from being known as a thief and a liar to being known as a man of integrity, an employee who has rarely been late or missed a day of work, and a person who has compassion for others. It's what has created within me a strong sense of character. Have you heard that term? Character is fundamentally a set of principles and values we live by, that we do not compromise, which gives our lives depth, direction, and meaning.

We don't see results overnight. When we plant an apple seed, we don't see the tree pop through the soil the next day. Weeks can go by when we don't see anything. Then all of a sudden, boom! That green little stub shoots out from the soil and then, if all goes well, it grows slowly and steadily over time. Once that tree begins to grow, it takes years for it to mature to the point that it can bear fruit. For our purposes, that gradual but lasting transformation is our freedom.

I don't have all the answers on how to live a life free from the bondage of my own diseased thinking. No one does. But I do have experience using the 12-step program I learned in Narcotics Anonymous (NA), which were derived from these principles, to begin putting distance between me and the diseased thinking that trapped me in active addiction for so long. The Bible and NA got me started on a path that led me to reading and studying how life works and understanding which principles would lead me toward my life goals.

This path began that day in the chow hall in St. Louis. When I got angry, I stopped accepting the defeat of addiction. And when I stopped accepting defeat, I went to work on changing my direction. Now it's your turn.

Are you willing to take this program, and start applying these principles, to gain an understanding of how you can start living a life free from active addiction?

In this section, I will share my experience, strength, and hope. For me those came with the understanding and the application of the 12 principles, and I will show how important elements of my character developed as I continued to practice them.

When we change our thinking by understanding and following these principles, we become able to free ourselves from lifestyles that create negative results. These principles are not just for addicts grappling with addiction. Understanding and applying these principles will empower anyone to transform into a person of with high moral standards, which leads to living a better life. The greatest gifts I can give others are the tools they need to live a lifestyle of high moral character.

This program worked for me; it's worked for others I've coached; and it will work for you. Let's begin.

Chapter Four: Give Up

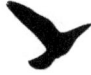

The spiritual principles that the 12 steps are derived from can be broken up into groups; each focuses on particular areas of character development. The three principles covered in this section are the basis of the first steps, which tell us to "give up," that is, we need to give up thinking we have control over our addiction and give in to the fact that it will be necessary to change some fundamental things about our lives in order to recover. The principles in this section are all focused on changing the thinking that we have control over our active addiction and figuring out how to become more responsible in our thoughts, actions, and behaviors. We are in control of our behaviors. God is not going to fix us. The power to change is within us. Because words can mean different things and can be open to interpretation, I am including the definition of what I mean at the beginning of each principle.

The Principle of Honesty
- *Honesty:* honor; honorableness; dignity; propriety; suitableness; decency.
- *Honesty:* the quality or state of being honest; probity; fairness and straightforwardness of conduct, speech, etc.; integrity; sincerity; truthfulness; freedom from fraud or guile.

Honesty is the antidote for diseased thinking, which makes it the first of the spiritual principles and the most important one. Everything we do is built on the foundation of honesty.

We have to be honest about our thoughts, words, and actions that led us to where we ended up. Only when we're honest can we face and break free from the captivity of active addiction.

There are situations, circumstances, and other people who introduce things into our lives that are beyond our control. We can't help that. We have to accept that. But we also have to understand what we can control.

We control how we respond to people and situations. We control whether our response is to walk out of that controlling situation, circumstance, or relationship quickly or slowly, or whether we walk away at all. We do this by being honest about the answers when we ask ourselves:

How is this situation affecting me?

How is this circumstance affecting me?

How is this person affecting me?

The *situation* could be that we have been involved with a group of people who are users and being in that situation makes it seem like using is okay.

The *circumstance* could be that we feel pain and regret for some of our actions, and we try to numb that pain by using.

The number-one *person* affecting us is ourselves. Honesty starts from within.

I was able to function for a long time when I was using. In the beginning, I could always figure out a way to get around the negative aspects of my using. Throughout my life, I was always able to think myself out of tough situations. But active addiction eventually had such a strong grip on me, it got to the point that I did not know how to handle my life anymore. Until I was honest about that, nothing was going to change.

Before going into that twelfth rehab, I hadn't been honest with myself or anyone else. Before that, I may have sort of acknowledged there might be a problem, telling family members I was going to quit soon but asking for $20 here and there to get high. I used to believe I was in control and that I could stop at any time. The twelfth rehab was when I finally started realizing what my problem was, and at long last started to understand what the solution might be.

I still remember so clearly sitting there all alone in the chow hall that day. I felt like a defeated man. I was in so much pain. Tears rolled down my face as I thought about how I was back in this situation again of being homeless, helpless, and penniless for the twelfth time, but now also 1,200 miles away from home. If I didn't get clean this time, it was surely going to be the end for me.

After letting myself feel that pain for a moment, I decided, "I'm here now and there's no need to feel sorry. I know what needs to happen. I just don't know how. I need to learn how to stop getting loaded and stay stopped."

My honesty that day was admitting to myself that I didn't know how to live. This private and personal moment of being honest with myself, of accepting the principle of honesty into my life, led me to take the first step of the 12-step program.

Step 1:
We admitted that we were powerless over our addiction,
that our lives had become unmanageable.

After all those years and all those rehabs, this was the first time I truly accepted the principle Step 1 is based on, and what it meant. I admitted that I didn't know how to free myself from the grips of active addiction, and that my "lives" had become unmanageable.

For a long time, I thought the second part of this step was talking about "we" as different people collectively realizing that our lives had become unmanageable. But I came to understand that this step was referring not to other people, but to all the parts of my existence affected by my using: my personal life, my business life, my married life, my financial life, my social life. All of this, all of these lives—*we*—had become unmanageable because of *my* powerlessness over addiction. Taking this step taught me that I was in this situation because of the decisions I made, period. It was not because of my uncles, my dad, or the jobs I'd had. It wasn't because of the people who sold me drugs or the people I did drugs with. It was because of *me*. I was the reason that I was in these situations, and I was responsible for all my lives becoming unmanageable. This important realization started me on the path to becoming open to learning how to live a lifestyle free from the use of drugs and alcohol.

When I looked at my failed marriage, my estranged daughters, my lost career opportunities, my homelessness—I saw a distinct pattern of bad habits. One habit that was common across the board was the blame game habit—my habit of laying the blame on anything and anyone but me. The blame game had to stop.

I had to let the past go. I had to let it go so I could grow, and what I needed was truth! Sitting at that table, I finally understood why I needed to practice the principle of honesty.

The first step is the only step we must do to the best of our abilities, every day. The rest of the steps are a work in progress, but in order for this program to work, we have to practice being perfect at being honest every day. We have to be brutally honest with ourselves and others on a daily basis, which means dealing with reality. We have to deal with things as they actually are and not be distracted by what we'd like for them to be or hope for them to be.

When I started working on perfecting the principle of honesty, I saw that I need to live each day based on the way my life is in that moment, at that exact point in time, and not dreaming about how I hope my life could be on any given day.

After the earlier treatment programs, I would get clean for a while. But then stinking thinking would kick in. I would tell myself, "Instead of smoking $100 worth of crack today, I'm only gonna get a $20 piece. I can handle that."

I couldn't handle that.

I told myself, "This time it won't control me. Nothing can control me."

Except that active addiction did control me.

"And I'm not going to land back in another treatment center."

Except that's where I landed time and again, because I could not be honest with myself. I still believed I had control over addiction; I did not accept and admit that addiction had control over me. I didn't know how to handle what I was feeling. Getting high was the only way to stop the voices.

Using allowed me not to feel, which was the only tool I had to make the pain go away. Whenever I felt pain over the loss of my daughters, of letting my nana down again and again, of doing harm to anyone I loved, including myself, I hit the crack pipe, and I didn't have to think about what I had done anymore. The crack brought me to an altered state of mind where I didn't see the issues that created the pain, and it temporarily took the pain away.

To my mind, I was going to manage using. Using was not going to manage me. That was the plan, but the plan never worked.

So many mornings after, I would tell myself, "I'm not getting high today." I had overdone it the night before. I had stayed out all night, then come home at four or five o'clock in the morning, dragging and beaten down. I hadn't eaten or sometimes even bathed for days.

I can remember looking at myself in the bathroom mirror and telling myself, "I can't keep doing this." Then I'd go to sleep and wake up at maybe two or three in the afternoon.

At around five or six in the evening, when it started getting dark, I would begin to get this feeling in my gut of wanting to get loaded, but I'd also think about what I had done the night before. That memory created pain, so I had to medicate that pain away, and this need gave me all the excuse I needed to get loaded again and again, day after day, night after night. It was like this thing would kick in my stomach, obsession, and a chain reaction would begin, a compulsion; this urge that I didn't know what to do with other than to feed it. And it was off to the races again. Whatever I'd told myself before going to sleep, whatever I'd promised myself in the morning, that was over. The urge to use overpowered everything. That lifestyle was hell, but I did it to myself over and over and over and over again.

I can remember at one point, when I was still working, I would try very hard to be responsible with my paycheck. I pulled out envelopes and labeled them so I could divide my money for my bills. I'd say, "Okay, this one's for my rent money, this one's for the electric bill, this one's for food, and this one's for cigarette money." Then I'd take $40 and set that to the side, telling myself, "This is all I'm taking to get high with this week. The rest of my check is going to pay bills."

I would separate out the money like this every Friday evening when I got paid. By Saturday morning, you know what happened to ALL the money, right? I smoked it up! All of it. I did that week after week after week. On Monday mornings, I went to work broke. No money for food, no money for cigarettes. Just broke in my wallet, and even more so, broke in my spirit. Yet I'd make it to work every day, even outperforming most of my peers. Despite the fact that I'd smoked up my entire paycheck in a couple of days.

My whole life revolved around using, a vicious cycle where addiction caused me to do things and make decisions that really weren't true to my nature or my heart. Almost every day, filled with pain and regret, I'd medicate away whatever it was I'd done to cause me pain the day before.

Finally, there came a time that I was no longer a *functioning* addict. I became a full-blown addict who used drugs to live, and I lived to use drugs. I lost my steady job and started hustling to keep some cash flowing. I still lied to myself that I was in control of using, but really, using was in control of me.

These days I don't lie to myself anymore, to the best of my ability. I'm not perfect. I can make mistakes like everyone else. But now I promptly admit when I'm wrong. I will not lie to Tim Stewart, because I've done it too many times before and it almost cost me my life.

So today and every day, I practice honesty with diligence. I look at my reality on a daily basis and make myself honest with my reality every day. I am an addict. I cannot use drugs. Because when I don't hold myself accountable for understanding and admitting this every day, I put my life back on the line.

I'm not confused about the danger of not being honest with myself. I've lived that horror flick. As I talked about earlier, I can remember looking in the mirror many mornings after coming in from a long night of getting loaded. The image I saw reflected back at me showed me my exact reality: a defeated human unable to break free from the bondage and grip of active addiction. Mirrors don't lie.

I was so miserable, I no longer wanted to live. This was the reality of my life and I had to face it. I had to admit I was an addict. My addiction controlled me. My lives as a son, grandson, husband, father, employee, had become unmanageable, and I had to do something about it.

I'm asking you to take a look in the mirror. Do you like the person you see? What are the things you like about this person? What about this person changes when you're using? Are you honest with others about what you're using? If not, why do you think you're hiding the truth?

EXERCISE #1: COME CLEAN

They say the journey of a thousand miles starts with a simple step. So the first exercise in the book to start you on your journey to recovery is one simple step. To complete this step, write down these words right on the page here so that when you come back to this page, seeing your words in your own handwriting will remind you that you and you alone were able to take this important step:

I AM AN ADDICT.

Once you admit it to yourself, once you commit it to writing that you have a problem, you are now being honest with yourself. Now you can begin the recovery process.

_____

_____

_____

_____

_____

_____

_____

_____

The Principle of Hope

- *Hope*: to desire with expectation of obtainment or fulfillment.
- *Hope*: to expect with confidence.

Remember that moment I told you about when I was sitting in the chow hall, and I realized how angry I felt? I balled up my fists, hit the table, and asked, "God, why? Why do I keep doing this to myself? Why do you keep letting this happen to me?" And do you remember that afterward, I felt as though God himself had spoken to me? In that moment, I didn't feel alone anymore.

I grew up in the church. My nana was a woman of God and would often tell me how God spoke to her. I had never had an experience like that before, but in that chow hall, I believed God was speaking to me because I had no other context to compare it to. Over time, I would come to accept that the voice was simply my inner voice, a power that lived within me and guided me when I stopped to listen to it. However, in my twelfth rehab, that voice and that belief in a higher power gave me the hope I needed to be able to take the second step.

Step 2:
We came to believe that a Power greater
than ourselves could restore us to sanity.

Step 2 is about the principle of hope. The hope that something bigger and more powerful than ourselves is able to bring us out of active addiction and into a place of positive habits and behaviors, so we can live clean and sober in a lifestyle of morality and sanity.

That's the good kind of hope. What I learned in taking this step is that we can always hope, but that hope can either be healthy or unhealthy.

What is unhealthy hope? Here's an example. When I was in New York, I'd put my money through a hole in a door on some city street at two in the morning, where I hoped that a runner would be there to bring my money to a dealer and bring me back some crack. I would randomly put my money in the hand of a person I could not see, with the unhealthy hope that they'd come back and bring me the hit I was craving and had paid for. Many times, I hoped the dude didn't just take my money and take off, which had happened on several occasions. That was the worst waiting experience on planet Earth, or at least it was for me at the time. Once he came back and I took that hit, I then hoped that hit of crack would take away the deeper pain of all the failures and hardships in my life. I hoped, and for a brief moment it did. In other words, I had an unhealthy hope that crack would relieve my suffering—when in actuality, what it was doing was causing my suffering.

So that's a way to live by hope, but it's definitely not the right way to live by hope. In this case, my hope was misplaced and misused, as I had hope in substances that never helped me with my problems. If anything, they only created more. Using enabled me to bury my problems. By getting high, I was stuffing my feelings, as we say in the program, instead of exposing them, dealing with them, and healing from them. Remember, I'd developed this coping mechanism from a very early age.

While I wasn't seeing it, relying on it, or using it in any positive way, healthy hope also started in the darkest days of my active addiction. I lived with my nana and granddaddy John (not the wealthy farmer grandfather) on and off during some of my most self-destructive years in active addiction, and my nana never gave up on me. She gave me hope, even if I didn't see it at the time. When everyone in Nana's life—her family, friends, and fellow Evangelist churchgoers—said, "Put him out! Cleo, you gotta put him out," she refused. She always told them, "I'm not putting him out because Jesus didn't let me go, and I'm not letting him go."

My nana was not happy with my lifestyle. She would rail me all the time for all my misdeeds and misconduct. But then she'd end her shouting tirades with, "God's gonna bring you out!" And then, something even more important. "You know I love you, don't you?"

Those days, as I said, I'd get home at dawn—and that was if I even made it home. Sometimes I'd stay on the street for days at a time, and I'd steal wallets and valuable items so I could buy more crack. Sometimes I'd even steal things from my grandparents' house.

They had an air conditioner in the kitchen window, and I saw it as something I could sell to get crack. Not my house. Not my air conditioner. But I took that air conditioner out of their kitchen window one day when they were out. I could only carry the thing about ten or fifteen feet before

I had to put it down because it was so heavy. But I managed to carry it out of their house and all the way down to the dope man. This was a very vivid example of the power of the obsession component of addiction.

When I finally came down from my high later that day, I felt so embarrassed about what I'd done, I hid in the closet. I just sat there with the door closed for hours—a grown-ass man sitting on the floor in the closet like a scared little child.

When they got back, they started calling out my name. Eventually my granddaddy found me in the closet. He opened the door and said, "Cleo, here he is."

And that was it. They didn't talk to me about the air conditioner. They knew I was the one who took it. They just accepted it. They said, "Okay," and they went out and bought a fan. The next time they went out, I took the fan out of the window and sold it to the dope man for another hit.

The only two people on the planet who let me live with them, and this is what I did to them. I explained earlier that active addiction is diseased thinking. It was truly a sickness.

It wasn't just crack that was my issue. I was so hooked on alcohol that I would drink Listerine right out of their medicine cabinet to get a fix from the high alcohol content. My granddaddy even marked the bottles to see how much I was drinking.

I not only felt like a lowlife, I *was* a lowlife. Still, my nana worked to give me that healthy hope, telling me over and over, "God's gonna bring you out." Nana's message of hope was one of the key rays of hope that made me give rehab another shot.

Another key ray of hope for me was the NA meetings I had previously attended. Despite not sticking with sobriety, I had gleaned some useful tips. During the meetings, we celebrated clean-time birthdays, and we had key tags to represent how long we'd been clean. Sometimes, when I was sitting there with a key tag for one or two days clean, and somebody walked in to get their key tag for having thirty days, sixty days, ninety days, a year, or even ten years clean, that gave me hope like you could never imagine.

In many meetings we get hope shots. A hope shot is when someone makes a comment on how they overcame a situation, and because the situation is similar to one you may be dealing with, and because it's something they overcame, you get a hope shot. We hear someone share the same problem, and we learn what they did to overcome that problem. Hearing that gives us hope that if a person overcame the same thing we're struggling to overcome, then there's hope we can overcome it too. A hope shot.

Once I got honest with myself, I was no longer attending meetings as a casual, skeptical spectator. I had finally accepted that I needed this treatment to live, and I began truly listening to how other addicts from all walks of life were now able to live their lives without using dope.

I was sick. People go to the hospital when they're sick, and I went to St. Mary's Hospital in St. Louis every Thursday night and Saturday afternoon to attend meetings. I attended other meetings and appointments during the week, but these two were mandatory. I especially liked the all-men's meeting on Saturday because I could really relate to their stories. Now I was focused. I was listening. I was sharing. This became an exciting new way of life for me. I found hope in learning how to stay clean.

Others at the meetings were dealing with life, one day at a time. One day at a time, one step at time, they were able to free themselves from themselves.

I realized that I had to replace my hope in dope with the hope that I could live a life without using. Believing "that a Power greater than ourselves could restore us to sanity" is what helped me begin to restart my life on a healthy path of hope. After I got honest with myself about how unmanageable my life had become, and how powerless I was in trying to fix it on my own, I now understood I didn't have to deal with my addiction on my own. Now I had the hope that this new Good Orderly Direction was going to help me get out of a lifestyle of unmanageability.

There's a saying: "We can only keep what we have by giving it away."

Today, I keep hope alive by constantly working to better myself and by sharing my story with other people to give them their hope shot like my nana, the NA program, and other recovering addicts have so freely done for me. I keep my hope by sowing hope into other people's lives.

I live with hope every day, and every day I have to choose (it's still a choice) to live in hope that the principles my Higher Power created will continue to help me restore my thinking in order to live the life I'm meant to live from the day I was born. Each hope shot I receive and give helps sow the grass seed in the soil of my soul so thick that the weed seeds can't take root.

Do you have someone in your life, like my nana, who gives you hope? Is there anything in my stories so far that gives you that hope shot you need to start freeing yourself from yourself? It all starts with our thinking.

EXERCISE #2: BELIEVE IN WHAT CAN BE

Having hope means being able to paint a picture in your head of what you want your life to look like. You have to be able to say to yourself, "I don't have to live this way. I don't have to continue on this path." And when you accept that truth, then it's time to ask, "What path do I want to be on?" This may sound strange, but until you become angry with who you are, you can never become who you want to be.

For the first part of this exercise, I want you to sit back and think. Take a good, hard look at your life and ask yourself if this is all you see for yourself.

Now I want you to focus on the good—or what could be good in your life if you are willing to change to achieve this life. What would your life look like if you could just have your life the way you wanted it to be?

Start with where you live. What would you change?

Look at who you know. Are these the people you would be connected to if your life looked exactly the way you wanted it to look?

Look at how you live your life, day to day. In the ideal version of your life, what would you be doing?

On this page, list ten things you want out of life. These could be material acquisitions, like buying a house or a new car. Or they can include things like finding a new love or starting a family. Seeing what you want written out on paper will bring you closer to achieving them. Instead of having your ideas and desires floating around, when you write them down it makes them more like a map or a guide.

TOP 10 THINGS I WANT IN MY LIFE

_____

_____

_____

_____

_____

_____

_____

_____

_____

_____

_____

_____

_____

_____

_____

_____

_____

_____

_____

_____

_____

_____

_____

_____

_____

_____

_____

_____

_____

Keep turning back to this list of goals with the hope that someday you can achieve them. You can start to make these things happen today, and as you continuously strive toward your goals, your hope will help carry you through to where God intended you to be.

The Principle of Faith

- *Faith*: allegiance to duty or a person; fidelity to one's promises; sincerity of intentions.
- *Faith*: belief and trust in and loyalty to God; belief in the traditional doctrines of a religion; firm belief in something for which there is no proof; complete trust.
- *Faith*: something that is believed especially with strong conviction, especially a system of religious beliefs.

The word *faith* comes from *pistis*, (PEES-tees) the Greek word for "faith," which means "firmly convinced."

When we talk about faith in this book and in the Free Yourself From Yourself program, we're not talking about a kind of blind faith that God's going to bless us with a car or something like that. Faith is not about expecting magic or miracles. It's about being able to believe something is true because we've had evidence that it is true. It's about having a clear and firm understanding of the spiritual principles and putting them into practice.

Faith is what we believe when we understand cause and effect—that an action will yield an anticipated result. For example, we're firmly convinced that when we go to work, our employers are going to pay us. We're firmly convinced that because we paid the electric bill, the lights will come on when we flip the switch. We're firmly convinced that when we sit down on a chair, it's going to hold us up. When we talk about faith, we're talking about that kind of faith—the faith based on laws and principles. I needed *faith* in the application of the principles found in the 12-step program's ability to teach me a new way to live.

In my recovery, I have learned that everything on this planet was created by and functions through laws, otherwise known as principles. Principles and laws are the same, except that principles focus more on the moral aspect of laws. This universe could not function if it did not operate by laws. My faith is that the laws are consistent; my faith is the framework for my morality.

Faith means different things to different people. The Bible defines faith as the substance of things hoped for and the evidence of things not seen. My faith comes when I have knowledge and understanding. I don't knock people for having this biblical definition of blind faith, as they call it, but my faith comes when I apply these principles. Today, my Higher Power is not some "guy in the sky" guiding my way. It is Good Orderly Direction. My faith is not in my imagination; my faith is based on tangible results produced from principles and laws.

When I first started out, I didn't understand this concept. I didn't know how to apply this principle. My Higher Power is different today than it was when I first went into recovery. At that time, because of the influence of my nana and other family members, I understood things through the lens of various Christian beliefs.

In the chow hall that day, my sense of morality was gone. My spirit was crushed. I had nothing to believe in. But then I received this message that God had delivered to me. I got up from the table. My tears dried up. Even my walk up to my room felt different. My steps felt lighter, but also purposeful. I had received the message that I had needed to hear twenty years ago. That message made me finally get honest with myself about how the results in my life had proved that I didn't know how to live.

God created these laws; it's up to us to discover and apply them. Sir Isaac Newton did not create gravity. He discovered it and shared his discovery so that others could understand. God doesn't make us act on spiritual principles. We act on them to become moral people.

From that point on, my focus changed. I looked around my room at the rehab center. I had a clean, private room with pictures on the walls. The bed was made tight. A lamp sat on the dresser. I noticed all those little things that people would take for granted if they hadn't come from a homeless shelter like I had. This room was like heaven for me compared to where I came from. I was starting to feel real hope, which is an important lead-in to faith.

I had faith, a productive kind of faith, for a few reasons now. For one, I had faith because Nana had always told me God would bring me out. I knew from clean-time stories shared in past NA meetings I had attended that life without using was real and possible. And now, adding to that, I believed God had just spoken to me.

When I found the Bible in the drawer, that excited my hope and my faith even more. Now I was ready to learn and I was going to read this Bible from beginning to end to learn how to live.

When I got to Genesis 1:11, "And God said, 'Let every seed produce after their own kind,'" I heard the voice again. I can still remember it like it was yesterday. After I read that, the voice said: "Words and deeds are just like seeds, they always produce after their own kind."

As I sat there, I thought about being back on the farm, remembering how seed, time, and harvest worked. Every time we planted a particular type of seed, that was what we harvested; each kind of seed produced a specific type of harvest. Every time.

I then said to myself, "This is a truth I can roll with. This is a fact, a tangible principle." I could understand faith in this way. Not as a person who had to believe in pie in the sky, but rather as a concept I fully understood, accepted, and already believed in: seed, time, and harvest.

I put my faith in the instructions written in the Bible, and that got me started on this step.

Step 3:
We made a decision to turn our will and our lives over
to the care of God as we understood Him.

The phrase "as we understood Him" is important. I didn't understand God the same way Nana did. She ate, slept, and breathed Jesus Christ. She always went to church or listened to sermons on the TV and radio. I grew up in a Baptist church in my small town with my parents, and I also attended Nana's Pentecostal church in Newark when I visited her every summer. These church experiences were quite different. They read the same book, but they worshipped in a completely different way. Despite my exposure to these church settings, I didn't have a real understanding of God at all. I came to understand, accept, and practice religion, but I did not know God. My understanding of God began to develop from that moment in the chow hall, when I received the revelation that I wasn't alone, which became the foundation of my recovery.

As human beings, we make decisions based on the information we receive or the environments we are subjected to. During my twelfth rehab, I came to realize that I was living and making decisions based on stories and information I'd received while growing up on the farm. Not the lessons of seed, time, and harvest, but the things I was learning and absorbing while I was hanging out with the farmhands and other older people—when I was replicating their habits because they were the only habits I knew.

In this twelfth rehab in St. Louis, I was starting to see that those things I'd absorbed and learned were no longer true for me. I'd been making decisions based on bad information and the results were bad. Feelings of pain and loss that were not properly processed had led to full-blown addiction. Making those bad decisions I'd landed sleeping on the floor of a homeless shelter hundreds of miles away from family and friends and living a defeated existence.

"Words and deeds are like seeds; they always produce after their own kind" became the foundation of my newfound faith. These words gave me a brand-new operating system for the way I would begin to live my life. I had finally received the right information from my Creator that would change my life forever and for the better.

As I mentioned earlier, we all have this kind of faith based on laws and principles. For example, when we get in the car and turn the ignition, we have faith that the car will start, because we know we put gas in the tank. The key to recovery is in learning to use that same kind of faith—faith in what is real and tangible—to replace old ways of thinking. The key is to choose ways of thinking that promote the growth of healthy lawns that choke out the weeds. Like in the landscaping example I shared with you in the first part of this book, we need to seed faith within ourselves, with new information and stories that lead to rich, bountiful harvests and that create good, strong habits and behaviors.

I needed *faith* in the application of the principles found in the 12-step program's ability to teach me a new way to live. Today, I continue to seek knowledge as I continue to be open-minded and learn from others. I'm still learning because, for me, faith is an equation: knowledge + under-standing = application. Even if I don't fully understand something, when

I have some knowledge, I can then have some faith and the results are the proof I'm seeking that lets me know I am on the right track.

Because I made that initial decision to use the Bible as a manual and instructions on how to live, and because I learned and practiced these important spiritual principles, I've harvested much better fruits in my life. The information and stories I relied on back when I was in active addiction, the weeds, are now choked out with positive new seed.

What do you think of when you hear the term "Higher Power?" Do you feel ready to start having faith based on things that are tangible, and concepts that are explainable? Are you ready to start seeding your belief?

EXERCISE #3: SEED YOUR BELIEF

Faith is something you have to actively work at having and maintaining. The Bible says, "Faith without work is dead." *Only if followed by action*, a belief or hope will equal faith. Taking actions or steps toward a goal is what faith is.

This exercise is not a writing exercise for the book; however, there is an empty page here for you to make notes on how you felt "testing your faith" by performing these quick and easy actions. Remember: the idea here is to approach an action with the understanding of what the result will be, because the principles of the universe make it so.

- Turn a light switch on and off—it was dark and now it's not.
- Turn on the water faucet in your kitchen—the water was off and now it's not.
- Wipe down your counter with a sponge—the counter was dirty and now it's not.
- Pour cereal into a bowl—the bowl was empty and now it's not.
- Pour orange juice into a glass—the glass was empty and now it's not.
- Brush your teeth—your mouth felt unclean and now it doesn't.
- Put on a sweater—you were cold and now you're not.

Think of some other basic causes that you know will produce an expected effect and act them out. The more you do this, the more you will have faith, and the more you will enforce for yourself, so that your actions will produce the results you want.

_____

_____

_____

_____

_____

_____

_____

_____

_____

_____

_____

_____

_____

_____

Chapter Five: Own Up

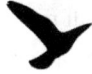

You've taken the first steps toward realizing active addiction is not something you can control on your own. You have a vision for what a clean and sober, successful life looks like, and you are working to establish a fundamental belief that if you act in a certain way, you can get the results you seek. You are on your way to experiencing what your life can be without drugs, alcohol, or any other compulsion that's been dragging you down. Now you're ready to learn about the next set of principles and take the next series of steps. This chapter encourages you to "own up." That means taking a good hard look at how active addiction has been harming your life, and how to start thinking, acting, and behaving differently in ways that get you closer to the person you are meant to be.

The Principle of Courage

- *Courage*: mental or moral strength to venture, persevere, and withstand danger, fear, or difficulty.

It takes a lot of courage to accept and admit that certain things we thought we knew about how to live haven't worked for us, that they'll never work for us, and to come to the understanding that we now have to unlearn and then relearn how to live. It can be very scary.

So many people are stuck living unhealthy, unproductive, unfulfilled, and defeated lives because they don't have the knowledge and courage to change. Change can be challenging and scary. If we let go of what we have known up to now and what has brought us this far, then what are we left with? We are left facing the unknown.

The 12 steps, and the principles they're derived from, are in a certain order because they are building blocks. For me, and for anyone else, I first needed to become *honest* about my lives being unmanageable. Then, I needed *hope* to believe that my lives didn't have to remain unmanageable. Finally, I needed *faith* that I could find a new way to live.

With the discovery of these principles in place, I worked to muster up the *courage* I needed to allow change to kick in. I could now let go of the bad information I had relied on all my life and grab hold of the program, the spiritual principles, and the people who were just like me to create the changes I needed to make in my lives.

That day in the chow hall, I felt like a poor pitiful nothing. I had to accept the first three steps. I had to give up. Then it became time to start owning up.

Courage is the start of owning up to everything I have been and everything I had caused to this point, and then focusing forward, moving to become a more morally grounded person, one day at a time.

When I had this new "design for living," I could free myself from myself with the understanding that every choice counts.

Step 4:
We made a searching and fearless moral inventory of ourselves.

I call myself a coach and a sponsor, and here's the reason. In the program, a sponsor is someone who has worked the 12 steps and becomes a guide to others as they work through them. I've sponsored many recovering addicts. As a life coach, I teach people how to handle complex life situations and circumstances. Personal relationships, difficult work environments, and addiction are examples of complex situations that are typically baffling, and if not handled properly, can lead to destructive behavior.

Many of us have baggage we're unable to face or handle alone, and sponsorship, the backbone of the program, definitely helps with handling the baggage. In the program, we frequently say that "the therapeutic value of one addict helping another is without parallel."

When I started out, I didn't know the heft of my baggage and how deep those bags were packed—that is, how deeply I had stuffed down my feelings into them. I knew I was broken, busted, and disgusted. I had lost everything—in terms of relationships and possessions, at least. But I didn't realize that I was carrying around baggage, which included some unresolved issues, harmful perspectives, and learned emotional responses from my past.

When I got to this step with my sponsor, I learned a lot about myself. He had me take a pen and a piece of paper and write out what I believed were my assets and my liabilities. This was not only to show what I needed to fix about me (liabilities) but also to show myself that I was not all bad—that there was still some good in me (assets).

At first, I had a hard time coming up with these assets. But, as time went by, they began to surface. For one, I knew I was pretty smart. I could speak well, and I could write pretty well. I was also a very loving and caring person. My grandmother said she stopped letting me take my toys with me to the playground when I was a little boy because I would always give them away to the other kids.

In the US Air Force, I'd done well at anything I put my mind to. I remember one time when I was deployed overseas, my Medevac unit landed in Beirut to rescue fallen soldiers. It was a gruesome scene. Not only were there bodies everywhere, but fingers and toes and other body parts were scattered everywhere. Doctors and nurses were passing out around me but I managed to stay focused. I had to intubate one woman. I was not a medical professional, but it was on me to put a tube down her throat and save her life. I had never done anything like that before, but we did what we had to do to save lives. And she lived! It gave me such a sense of accomplishment and gratitude to be able to save her like that. I felt like I had contributed; that I had created a solution in a disaster situation.

Can't was not a word in my vocabulary before active addiction took hold. I was often hired for jobs that required degrees, despite my not having any degrees. I think this was because I was a very confident person and a good salesman and my military background carried a lot of weight.

I added these assets to my list over time. By working with my sponsor, being in the program, attending meetings, and hanging out with other recovering addicts, I was eventually able to see the good within myself. But it did not happen overnight. I didn't become addicted in one day, and my recovery was not going to happen in one day. However, as I began to understand and practice the principle of "every choice counts," one day at a time, my life was changing for the better. I started to feel good about being alive again. My walk got some of its swagger back.

In order to complete this step properly, I also had to list my liabilities: I had been dishonest at times, mostly with myself. I was a disappointment and an embarrassment to my family. I had no contact with my daughters. I was disconnected. I was a miserable human being from all the pain and loss, and I often self-medicated.

It took courage to look at these liabilities and choose which ones I would work on first, but having the assets listed alongside them helped me to see I wasn't all bad, and that if I worked at it, I could have a longer column of assets than of liabilities. In building courage, I no longer felt morally bankrupt. I became less and less afraid to take suggestions from my sponsor and from people who had been on this path much longer than I had.

As I continued to build up this spiritual principle of courage, one day at a time, I began adding up some days of clean time, and I was less afraid, because I was beginning to see positive results, both external and internal: I could keep a job. I had a car. As I worked through this step, I was able to evaluate clearly those areas of my character that needed the most help and start working on them.

I found out that just like there's the bad kind of hope, there's the bad kind of courage. In the past I had used my courage to produce some pretty negative results. While I was in active addiction, I relied on courage to travel up and down the highways with illegal drugs. I relied on courage to sell drugs and hang out with some dangerous people. What I believed at the time to be my best thinking and decisions had landed me in some terrifying situations, but now, by relying on the right kind of courage, the results were very different.

In recovery, I had to channel courage differently. I had to find good courage and turn it to listening and adopting the suggestions of others who had once lived as captives like me, but now lived the lifestyle I wanted to live.

Even today, I continue to take suggestions and practice this principle of courage on a daily basis. Writing this book, running the Free Yourself

From Yourself program, and sharing my personal story in this way, all requires a great deal of courage.

What activities are you currently engaging in that require courage? How can you channel your courage to produce positive results in your life? Do you know someone who was once held captive by the same way of thinking as you, and is now free? What suggestions do you think they could offer that you can adopt right now, today?

EXERCISE #4: TAKE A MORAL INVENTORY

It's time for you to take a moral inventory of your assets and liabilities. This will be one of the hardest exercises in the book, but I promise it will also be the most important one you'll do, and one you'll keep referring to and updating for years to come.

Take a sheet of paper and draw a line down the middle. Or use the table below for this exercise. Notice there are two columns on this table. The left-hand side reads ASSETS; the right-hand side is LIABILI-TIES. Take a pen and start writing down assets and liabilities under these headers. Don't take time to reflect; just start writing whatever comes to your mind for the next fifteen minutes or so.

ASSETS	LIABILITIES

ASSETS	LIABILITIES

Now look at what you wrote down. How can you get the things you listed in your assets column to outnumber your liabilities column? Keep reading.

The Principle of Integrity

- *Integrity*: firm adherence to a code of especially moral or artistic values.
- *Integrity*: an unimpaired condition.
- *Integrity*: the quality or state of being complete or undivided.
- *Integrity*: doing what you mean and meaning what you say.

Honesty and integrity may sound similar, but they are different. Honesty simply means telling the truth, while integrity means living a lifestyle according to a set of personally enforced strict ethics—being honest in all of our activities, personal as well as business, when no one's looking as well as when you're being watched. Honesty can be a onetime event, yet when I tell the truth and get honest repeatedly, day after day, week after week, it becomes part of how I live. It becomes my character, and when I constantly use it as my tool for making decisions and dealing with myself and others, I become a person of integrity.

The Bible describes the word *holiness* as a state of being that occurs when one's words, thoughts, and actions are the same, and this is at the core of the meaning of integrity. You can't think one thing, say something else, and do yet another thing and still obtain holiness.

My words, my thoughts, and my actions are integrated, and this empowers me to live a lifestyle of integrity. No real and lasting success in life comes without the understanding and application of the spiritual principle of integrity. No matter the lifestyle or business, integrity must be the foundation.

The practice of integrity allows me to live with a clear conscience and be consistent, so I'm the same person at one o'clock in the afternoon as I am at one o'clock in the morning. I'm not a different person on Monday than I am on Sunday. I'm pretty much the same in my personal and professional lives.

Living a lifestyle of integrity is a choice, and as you now know, every choice counts. The practice of integrity means we don't do sneaky stuff that's gonna come back to bite us in the butt and cause us pain, because we know that pain and shame gives us that urge to self-medicate with drugs, alcohol, sex, gambling, or another addictive habit. But one little compromise away from integrity greases the wheel for the next. Like other things we try for the first time, it's harder at first to live a lifestyle of integrity if this has not been our method of operation; however, it becomes easier with practice over time.

We may still make mistakes, but we can make sure our motives are never ill. If we make a mistake, it's an honest mistake, and we can admit that we made that mistake. We can replant the right seed and reap the right harvest. We can start anew.

Step 5:
We admitted to God, to ourselves, and to another
human being the exact nature of our wrongs.

This fifth step is about transitioning to a life of integrity where our thoughts, words, and lives align. To get there, we have to give voice to those times when we've wronged others. When we admit to wrongdoing and strive to make amends, we clear the way for a new life of integrity. We start by making amends to ourselves. We build to being able to make amends to others.

I have been through all 12 steps and practiced their basic principles for more than sixteen years. As I have been all the way through the program, I have a full awareness of when I've done something wrong and what I need to do to correct it. This may not be obvious to you at first. It takes time.

These days, if I do something at home that I shouldn't have done, or if I say something to my wife that maybe I shouldn't have said, I'll immediately make amends. It's not always easy to do, but it's essential to living a lifestyle of integrity. It's far easier to do what's right than to undo a wrong, but admitting wrong goes a long way.

It's going to take you some time to get to the place where you can see that you've done something that goes against the principle of integrity, and that's okay. You're just getting started on this path. The more you learn—about the principles, yourself, and your place in the world—the more these situations will become readily apparent for you.

Saying what I mean and meaning what I say is integrity in its purest definition. Tim Stewart holds Tim Stewart accountable, and this, my dear friends, has become my character and my lifestyle. For me, my very life depends upon it.

Practicing a lifestyle of integrity can be difficult at times, because we also may expect others to also live with integrity, and so many people do not live that way. My feelings have been hurt many times for striving to do the right things to the best of my ability, while others are okay with not living a lifestyle of integrity. That's their choice. Sometimes my family members maintain their distance from me because when they call and ask my opinion, I must tell them truth instead of saying what they may want to hear. I must tell them truth because I know how operating with truth made me free from myself.

John 8:32 in the King James Bible states it this way: "And ye shall know the truth, and the truth shall make you free."

If I fail to tell people what I know to be true, then I can't say, fully and with all honesty, "I love you" to that person, and mean it with the greatest level of authenticity. I can believe what I want about a person and base my love for them on what I want to see, but that's not integrity. To really and fully love a person (including myself), I have to take a look at how things are and not sweep it under the rug. I have to fully understand and accept the reality, and I have to love on those terms. If my wife says something that hurts my feelings, I have to tell her in that moment, "You hurt my feelings." And I have to fully accept her response to that statement. I continue to love her, knowing that her response shows me who she is, and I accept her response, knowing that she is who she is and not who I want her to be. That's integrity.

We start by applying this principle to ourselves. Living with this level of integrity does not happen overnight. However, the daily practice of the principle of integrity has helped me free myself from myself and from the use of drugs and alcohol.

When I was using, I had become what one would call a professional thief in many areas of my life. I already told you about the air conditioner and the window fan I stole from my grandparents to pay for dope. That was when I was using, but I can't tell you in all truth that the mindset of being a thief just magically vanished when I stopped using.

I can remember once when I was two years clean and sober, after this twelfth rehab, that my wife and I wanted a DVR. We went into a well-known retail store to find one. She didn't know what I was up to at the time, but I put a DVR in a shopping cart and walked right out of the store without paying for it. That was not my plan when we went into the store, but that old mindset kicked back in, and suddenly, I saw it as an exciting challenge to steal the DVR.

What's my point?

As much as I strive to live a lifestyle of integrity today, meaning I don't steal, lie, or cheat, I can still slip up because I had lived an opposite lifestyle for so much longer than the one I'm living today. Even now, I can still be tempted to walk out of the store without paying for something. But then I play that scene all the way out in my mind; I could get caught or go to jail or be tortured by my conscience for giving in to temptation.

I say to myself, out loud if I have to, "No, I ain't doin' that today. I don't live like that anymore. It's not worth the consequences."

In 2 Corinthians, Paul tells us: "We take every thought captive and bring it into the knowledge and obedience of Christ." That's a direct instruction. King Solomon says in Proverbs, "So as a man thinketh, so is he." The Bible instructs that we are a product of our thoughts.

I practice controlling my thoughts by opening my mouth and speaking words that oppose any negative or destructive thoughts I have before I act on them. This exercise is called "capturing thoughts," and it helps people correct their thinking.

For example, I may notice an attractive young lady, and I may think I want to give her my number. Before I do, I capture my thought. I open up my mouth, and remind myself, "I am married. This idea I'm having of giving this other woman my number is wrong. That violates my covenant with my wife." Now I have captured that thought, and I have not acted on it. I may have to say it to myself ten times. You may have to say it to yourself ten times, or twenty—whatever it takes. But it's all about being accountable for our actions and behavior. And it becomes easier with time, when the joys and richness of the life of integrity are in the balance.

When I was in active addiction, I battled thoughts with thoughts. I didn't understand back then that words capture thoughts. I would think to myself, "I'm not getting high today." But I rarely opened my mouth and said it out loud. So, when the thought came for me to go get high, I hadn't captured it. I hadn't dealt with that thought. I hadn't put that thought into subjection, looked at it and said it and owned it. And so I got loaded.

So many times in my life I attempted to fight negative thoughts with positive thoughts, and most times the negative thoughts won. But "taking every thought captive" has helped me become much more honest with myself and others.

Try it yourself. The next time you're thinking about acting on something you know is maybe not the best thing you can be doing, tell yourself, out loud, that you should not be doing that:

"I should not be asking that woman for her phone number."

"I should not be wanting to take that wallet I found on the floor and pocket it for myself."

"I should not take that drink, as much as I want to have that drink, because that drink will only lead to more drinking—hurting myself and those I love."

I don't proclaim to be holier than thou. I still get bad thoughts. The difference is, because of integrity, now I don't act on them. Now, if I don't tell the truth, it will upset me, and I will be uneasy in my spirit, whereas prior to this new lifestyle, telling a lie was as easy as eating a slice of bread. When I practice this principle of integrity, I don't cause myself harm, physical or emotional, and therefore, there is no need to self-medicate.

Up to this point, we've talked about practicing *honesty*, which comes when we realize we don't have control over these addictive practices and behaviors and admit that we need help.

We talked about *hope* and getting those hope shots to inspire us to understand and believe that change is possible.

We explored the idea that *faith* that God, as we understand him, will help us experience the positive changes we need while we step through this program to a new way of living.

We learned about the *courage* we need to face the parts of our character we need to work on.

And now we've talked about how the practice of *integrity* helps us align our thoughts about who we are with how we talk and how we act, so that we are one.

Honesty becomes a lifestyle called integrity, and we learn to practice integrity for the same reason we take a bath—without it, we stink. As I mentioned earlier, living with integrity is not a onetime event. We constantly have to practice making the right choices, every moment of every day.

It is our responsibility to sow the right seeds thick by practicing these principles. By speaking the right words into our ears. By making sure our eyes are on what's right, pure, and true. We sow these integrity seeds so thick that when the thought of being dishonest comes up, the weed seeds of bad thought gets choked out by the lush growth of all the right seed thoughts.

As I continue to develop my character, I continue to live a lifestyle of integrity and morality. The greatest gift I can give myself is a lifestyle of integrity. The greatest gift I can give others is to be a model character for the benefits of living a lifestyle of integrity.

Do you try to do the right thing, even if the consequences of your actions won't benefit you? Do you speak up about your values, even if it might mean you don't get what you want? Are you ready to start doing what you say, and living each day practicing integrity? Are you willing to let go of trying to see things as you want them to be, and start seeing things as they are? Are you ready to take this next step, and commit to paper who you are—who you have been, and who you're ready to become?

EXERCISE #5: INTEGRITY INVENTORY

Living a lifestyle of integrity means living a life based on values that you hold and uphold, that you are unwilling to violate no matter what. On this page, answer the following true or false:

I am honest with others.   _____

I am ethical in personal dealings. _____

I am ethical in in business dealings. _____

I deliver on the promises I make. _____

I treat others fairly. _____

I don't ignore the wrongdoing of others. _____

I stick up for others. _____

To live a life of integrity, you should be able to answer all of the above in the affirmative. How many of these attributes were true for you? How many do you still need to work on? Feel free to take notes below.

_____

_____

_____

_____

_____

_____

_____

_____

_____

_____

_____

_____

_____

_____

_____

_____

_____

_____

_____

_____

_____

_____

_____

_____

_____

The Principle of Willingness

- *Willing*: inclined or favorably disposed in mind.
- *Willing*: prompt to act or respond.
- *Willing*: done, borne, or accepted by choice or without reluctance.
- *Willing*: of or relating to the will or power of choosing.

Once I started to have some clean time under my belt, and the more I continued to practice the principles that made these steps, the more I began to feel like I mattered—that I had a purpose for being here on planet Earth. I always wanted to believe I had a purpose in life, as most everyone does, but now I *knew* I had a purpose, because I was still *here*.

There were so many times my life could have ended, but it didn't. One day at a time, I no longer wanted to steal, because I didn't want the embarrassment of being a person who stole things, like the grown man who had cowered in his grandparents' closet after stealing from them. Instead, I wanted to become a person of high moral character, someone who could be trusted. I no longer wanted to live a lie. I wanted to be faithful, because I realized that the defects of my character could cause me to feel pain and then lead me down the path to using again, back to what I knew best: self-medicating, letting the weeds choke out everything good and useful that tried to grow.

Once I understood the work I had to do to become the moral person I wanted to be, I had to become willing to do the work. I discovered that God was not going to magically heal me; I had a part to play in this whole grand scheme of things. It's one thing to know what you have to do; it's another thing to commit yourself to going through with it. This is what the principle of willingness is all about.

The Bible, the 12-step program, and the philosophy that everything counts became the motivating tools I used to start doing the work to become a person of high moral value.

I came to trust the Bible as a manual filled with instructions on how to live here on this planet and how to operate as a human being. I found the formula for success in Joshua 1:8, which says, "This book of the law shall not depart out of thy mouth; but thou shalt meditate therein day and night, that thou mayest observe to do according to all that is written therein: for then thou shalt make thy way prosperous, and then thou shalt have good success."

This instruction for being successful rang loud and clear in my ear. If I wanted success, I had a part to play. Even though I did not fully understand at the time how it all worked, I discovered this scripture, which made it clear to me that my Creator had already helped me out of this lifestyle and would continue to do so if I did my part and followed the instructions.

It wasn't enough to understand the principles. I had to become *willing* to understand and apply them to my life. I had to be willing to trust that by the understanding and, most important, the active application of instructions written in this manual, my life would change—not by magic. I had to be willing to apply the principles I learned to help me remove the defects in my character that had led me to getting loaded time after time after time, even when I didn't want to.

I came to understand and accept the Bible as a manual, "the Maker's mind." What do I mean by that? Think of it this way. Manuals are booklets written by the manufacturers of products: "Hey, here's what I have put into this product. Here are the features and benefits of this product. Here's how you can use this product. And here's what you don't do with this product." In others words, these are the "laws" for this product.

The Bible contains the same kind of instructions, woven into stories that convey lessons of morality. The stories are there to give the principles context, but the principles are the actual instructions. The Bible shows the features of the product—the principles gleaned from the Bible stories. Then the Bible shows how to use these features, with stories that incorporate the principles to deliver the message of the Maker. In that way, the Bible is the Maker's mind.

In order to receive the message, I had to be willing to find the principles within the stories, and be *willing* to do the work to apply these principles to my life. I had always been taught and believed that God made me. Now, with this new, concrete understanding of the principles outlined in the Bible, I was willing to follow the instructions provided so that I could change.

Step 6:
We were entirely ready to have God remove
all of these defects of character.

It's not magic. You don't get zapped with the principles and all of a sudden, you're healed. It takes work. It takes a willingness to do the work. Before this step, we were discovering the concepts of recovery. This is where the rubber meets the road. In this step, with the principle of willingness guiding us, we actively start to do the work. We've put the tires on the car; now it's time to drive the car.

When I took this step, I became willing to practice these principles in the manual and the program, and I became willing to do the work I needed to do to create new habits. I understood that the only way my defects of character would go away was if I got rid of the bad habits and behaviors, and to do that, I had to change how I thought. The weeds would not just disappear on their own. My understanding of "God helping me" was all up to me being willing to follow these instructions and practice this program to the best of my ability.

I became willing to change these negative character defects, habits, and behaviors so I could live a higher quality of life. Today I am living that higher quality of life I desired for so long but just didn't know how to achieve. I made a commitment to develop healthy new habits, like the habit of being *honest* and telling the truth, of living a lifestyle firmly rooted and grounded in *integrity*. I was willing to open myself to let hope in, and to do the work to discover a foundation for faith. I was willing to have the courage to face who I had been, and start working toward the person I wanted to become. I also started to become *willing* to share my experience, strength, and hope with other people, which I will talk about in more detail as we move through the later principles and steps in this book.

A man dying of starvation can see a plate of food across the table from him, but unless he's willing to do the work, to walk across the room to get to that food and eat that food, he will drop dead. Knowing what to do is one thing. Being willing to act and do the work is something else. It's not enough to know we have character defects. We need to be willing to do the work to correct them.

Some people don't care about their lifestyle. They operate at a level of selfishness that blocks any remorse in how their choices hurt themselves or others. That used to be me, but I don't cheat, I don't steal, and I don't lie anymore. I try to be good to the best of my ability. No one is perfect, but I can honestly say that today I am a faithful man to myself, my wife, my employer, and whomever I do business with, because I became willing to allow my Creator to guide me in removing all my defects of character. I became willing to start practicing these principles, and this is what has made possible the life I live today.

Will we continue to tolerate the habits that bring to us and others around us hurt, harm, pain, and shame? Are we going to continue to tolerate a lifestyle of practicing negative habits? Or are we mad enough and frustrated enough that we are ready for change?

Ask yourself: Am I willing to do the work I need to do to remove all my defects of character?

EXERCISE #6: SET YOURSELF ON YOUR PATH

If you're not willing and ready to change, you're not going to change. It's really that simple. No one can spark change and set you on the right path except you. But to get on that path, you have to fully understand that this is about you doing what you have to do to change the conditions and landscape of your life. You have to be able to look at the current path you're on and get angry that you're not living a lifestyle of morality. You're not living the life you were always intended to live. You have to get mad enough about the way things are to change the way things are.

Setting out on this path isn't going to be easy, but it will become easier once you start walking it, taking it one day at a time.

Read these statements out loud, slowly and deliberately. Pay attention to each of the words as you speak them:

- I am willing to trust myself that I am good enough and that I deserve to live a good and moral lifestyle.
- I am willing to ignore those who may try to hold me back from starting to walk on this path, especially others I may be associating with who are in active addiction.

- I am willing to stay on this path, even if it means I'm on the journey by myself.
- I am willing to keep walking on this path, even if I don't see the results I want right away.
- I am willing to ask for help when I need it.
- I am willing to forgive myself without hating myself if I wander off the path—and I am willing to step back onto the path should I ever wander off.

This page will become a source of motivation for you as you continue on in your journey to recovery. At least once a week, if not more, come back to this page. Read these statements out loud. Keep repeating all the good information into your ear to choke out the bad information within you. I've left some space below in case you want to write notes on how these statements impact you.

_____

_____

_____

_____

_____

_____

_____

_____

_____

Chapter Six: Make Up

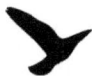

In the last section, called "Own Up," we took some important steps. Those steps and their defining principles had to do with looking within; we were taking a moral inventory of ourselves—our actions, habits, and behaviors—and understanding why what we had been doing was hurting us and keeping us from becoming the people God intended us to be when we were created.

Now it's time to deal with how your active addiction has affected others. Remember that active addiction has not only harmed your life, it has also taken a pretty big toll on your loved ones, your coworkers, and others you've interacted with. So, as we get closer to recovery, we'll work on healing some of the other damage your addiction has caused.

The Principle of Humility

- *Humility*: freedom from pride or arrogance; the quality or state of being humble.

The program tells us that having humility is as essential to keeping clean as food and water is to staying alive.

Before my twelfth rehab, I lacked humility. I was always a prideful person, but I had to get humble and allow someone else to teach me how to live. I had to humble myself and ask God to help me with my shortcomings. If I didn't humble myself, I knew that I would continue to be humiliated. Becoming humble didn't mean becoming weak. It meant I had to drop my pride from all areas of my life.

When I was in active addiction, I used to make "foxhole prayers." The term comes from when a soldier on a battlefield says a prayer from the foxhole, making a bargain with God to be spared. I prayed many of those from the streets: "Just get me out this one time, Lord! I won't do it again, I promise you. Just get me out of this one."

During some of my darkest days in active addiction, I would sometimes rent out my car to get money for crack. "Lord, if you make them bring it back, I promise I won't rent out my car to get drugs ever again!"

Another time, I got caught up in a raid. I was in a group, trying to see if we could score some drugs, and the cops came and arrested six of us. The other guys were already convicted felons and the prosecutor wanted to work out a deal with them regarding jail time. I had never been convicted of a crime, so the deal they were making wasn't going to work out for me. I would become a convicted felon. I didn't take the deal, and I had to go to court, where if I got convicted, I would have to do time—a mandatory five years. I prayed another foxhole prayer. "Please, Lord. Bring me out of this. Don't let them convict me and throw me in jail, and I will stop using."

I didn't get any time. In fact, I didn't even have to go to court, but of course, I didn't stop using. My rationalization this time? It wasn't my prayer God was answering. He'd answered my nana's prayer; and that's what everyone else thought, too.

But I finally realized, if I wanted to get better, I had to let go of the old ways. I had no more bargaining room. As I explained before, I grew up around money. My family had money. In fifth grade, I could be walking around with hundred-dollar bills in my pocket. I was working on the farm and in the stores, and I was also a thief. I was the boss of the staff. I made demands on anyone I pleased. But I had nothing when I landed out in St. Louis. I couldn't make demands on anyone. I had to humble myself and submit to the instructions of others.

To this day I practice humility as a choice, but back in that shelter, it wasn't my choice. That experience humbled me. At that shelter, I stopped making foxhole prayers. I knew I couldn't make any demands, because I had never held up my end of the bargain. From that point on, I started making humble prayers.

Step 7:
We humbly asked Him to remove our shortcomings.

When we humbly request God to remove our shortcomings, it can't be a foxhole prayer. When I took this step toward living the principle of humility, I had to forgive myself for some of the things I did. I had to first become humble in my own spirit, before I could start humbling myself to other people. Even today, I sometimes find myself reverting back to the person I was, and I have to catch myself. That's practicing humility.

Remember earlier, when I talked about Dr. Myles Munroe and his media principles? Our Creator gave us emotions but didn't give us these emotions for them to manage us. It's up to us to manage them. We manage our emotions through practicing humility. This is one of the biggest lessons I learned from Dr. Myles.

I had to replace the arrogance and pride that once defined me. Back in the day, people couldn't tell me I couldn't do something. Sometimes, I did things just to prove people wrong. If I decided to do something, I did it, no matter what. I guess that's why it took me twelve times before treatment stuck. For the first eleven times, I was just so determined that dope was not going to beat me. I was convinced, wrongly, that I could do dope and I could manage it, or that I could smoke crack and still live the lifestyle I wanted to live. The thing about addiction is that it's progressive. The more years I invested in that active addiction lifestyle, the more of a grip it had on me.

For a lot of people, humility doesn't come until they find themselves humiliated. That was my story. I was humiliated, living in a homeless shelter, sleeping on the floor, taking community showers. I felt beaten, but I knew I had to get up off the mat and fight another round. That was my motivation: I wondered how I could change my circumstances. First, I had to figure out some things about me. I had to listen to other people about who I was, and I needed to have a better awareness of who I was, especially when it came to my shortcomings. The way I had been fighting my addiction wasn't working, and I needed a fresh perspective.

I was always a fighter. In high school, I would fight on a dime to protect someone who was being bullied or otherwise wronged, just like Uncle Wiggy. Problem was, I could go from 0 to 100 in no time. Typically, before a fight broke out on school grounds, there was a back-and-forth dialogue that occurred, an escalation before the first punch was thrown.

There was no escalation process for me. If I had any idea there was going to be a fight, I made it a point to land that first punch, because Uncle Dave taught me that the one who lands that first punch wins. I lived by his words, and I didn't lose many fights. I wasn't walking around with a chip on my shoulder or anything like that, but if someone brought the business to me or to anyone else close to me, I handled the business. As a result, I got suspended from high school five times—ouch.

I didn't understand it at the time, but in fighting all the time like that, I was giving in to my emotions and my shortcomings. A shortcoming is the action tied to a character defect. In other words, when we act on a character defect, we end up with a shortcoming. Inflicting harm on another person because of a character defect leads to a shortcoming. My character flaw (self-centeredness) triggered my shortcoming (fighting to get attention). I rarely got any positive attention at home, except being asked if I had washed out all the turkey waters and finished all my other work. I was almost always in trouble, so I guess it was just hard for my parents to give me any positive attention. Anyway, I had a character defect, self-centeredness, but as soon as I hit someone, it became a shortcoming, which was fighting to get attention. Each time we give in to a shortcoming, it gets easier to give in to the next one.

There were many things I didn't know about myself over the years, for instance, that I had these character defects and shortcomings. I didn't realize it was not the drugs and the alcohol that brought me to where I landed, but a lot of unthinking reactions and behaviors all along the way. I didn't realize that the issue was deep within me, weeds that choked out most of the healthy, moral crops that needed to be there. Had I been able to get honest with myself much earlier in my life and realized that I could work on my character defects instead of medicating my pain, I would have saved myself and my loved ones a lot of years of pain and loss.

Humility is the result of getting honest with ourselves. Humility means examining character defects and working on character development. Here are the defects of character, as defined by Narcotics Anonymous (NA):

- Resentment, Anger
- Self-centeredness

- Fear, Cowardice
- Self-pity
- Self-justification
- Self-importance, Egotism
- Self-condemnation, Guilt
- Lying, Evasiveness, Dishonesty
- Impatience
- Hate
- False pride, Phoniness, Denial
- Jealousy
- Envy
- Laziness
- Procrastination
- Insincerity
- Negative thinking
- Immoral thinking
- Perfectionism, Intolerance
- Criticizing, Loose talk, Gossip
- Greed

I thought drugs and alcohol were the problem, but I was wrong. Because of pride (self-importance, egotism), I avoided doing the work on myself that needed to be done to make myself stop harming myself and others (shortcoming). I hadn't been honest with myself, hadn't admitted that the problem was within me. I thought I controlled the problem. That was my diseased thinking.

As long as I kept thinking that the drugs and the alcohol were the problem, I kept breaking the weed off at the top of the dirt and leaving the root to grow again. When God—or rather, the voice—revealed to me that my thinking was the problem, I started pulling weeds up by the root, and that's the only way to get rid of deeply rooted weeds. Because if we pull a weed up at the root, it's not coming back up; now we may get another one over to the side, to the right or to the left of it, but that one root is not coming back up again!

Are you ready to correct your shortcomings by discovering the character defects within you that trigger them? Are you willing to be honest with yourself and take responsibility for your shortcomings? Are you open to reaching out to your Higher Power for guidance as you work to correct the flaws that keep you from living clean and sober? Now let's do the work.

EXERCISE #7: ASSESSING SHORTCOMINGS

Turn back to the list you created in Step 4. What are some of the short-comings you wrote down here? List them in the column under the heading "Shortcomings."

You now understand that these shortcomings occurred as a result of character defects, also known as liabilities. Go back to the list of character defects we covered earlier. How many of the 21 character defects I listed above do you spot in your list? Can you connect any of them to one of your shortcomings? List those in the "Character Defects" column.

SHORTCOMINGS	CHARACTER DEFECTS

SHORTCOMINGS	CHARACTER DEFECTS

Now we ask our Higher Power for instructions, for help in removing our shortcomings. Remember, your Higher Power is who or what you want it to be, as long as it's loving and caring. It's not necessarily "the big guy in the sky." It's a power that guides you that's bigger than you. For me, it's the set of principles I live by. Whatever it is for you, work with your Higher Power to figure out what you can do to fix what's broken. And now, let's do something about it.

The Principle of Discipline and Action

- *Discipline*: control gained by enforcing obedience or order; orderly or prescribed conduct or pattern of behavior; self-control.
- *Discipline*: training that corrects, molds, or perfects the mental faculties or moral character.
- *Discipline*: a rule or system of rules governing conduct or activity.
- *Action:* a thing done; the accomplishment of a thing usually over a period of time, in stages, or with the possibility of repetition; behavior; conduct.
- *Action:* an act of will.
- *Action:* the bringing about of an alteration by force or through a natural agency.

In my life today, I am responsible when it comes to my family and my employer. I treat everyone with respect, and I do what I'm supposed to do. I eat right and I get proper rest so I can fulfill my responsibilities to the best of my abilities. This takes *discipline*, in knowing I have to stay the course and keep responsible, as well as *action*, in continuing to keep moving toward the healthy goals I set for myself. The more *disciplined* I am, the more I *act* to fulfill my commitments and meet my responsibilities, and the better results I get. The only bad thing about discipline is that it can be very easy to lose. Remember, one compromise greases the wheel for the next, so you have to keep on it.

I have spent the last seven years working in college admissions. I enjoy the work I do. I have a passion for it, and the work gives me a deep sense of purpose. I remember my first job in admissions. I started as a trainee with eleven others. I got promoted quickly. I was highly regarded for the effort I put in, and everyone was aware of the kind of job I was doing, including my higher-ups.

Unfortunately, some people in management started doing some things I didn't feel were ethical. I had no choice but to resign from the job. After I resigned, the CEO called me personally to find out what happened. Apparently, she had gotten wind of the situation that caused me to leave, and she offered to rehire me, promote me to a management position, and gave me a $10,000 raise. My discipline and action in performing that job had made such an impact, the big boss would not let me go.

While at that job, my work ethic was second to none. It was one of the positive character traits I'd developed from having worked on the farm all those years. I lived very close to that workplace. Whenever they were in a crunch, they'd call me, sometimes at the last minute or on my days off, to cover for others. I certainly couldn't help out on a moment's notice like that if I was still getting loaded. Because I was able to help whenever I could, I was valued at my job. I was disciplined to do the work. My character showed in the passion and commitment I demonstrated when I went to work.

Step 8:
We made a list of all persons we had harmed,
and became willing to make amends to them all.

In Integrity, we start by making amends to ourselves. In Discipline and Action, we now actively begin making amends to others.

I took action in rehab. I worked with my sponsor to write out the list of people I had wronged and to whom I needed to make amends. The people on this list included my nana and granddaddy John, my mom and my dad, my daughters, and my ex.

When I finished the list, I handed it over to him. He took a look at it and said, "I don't see your name on here."

I hadn't thought about the harm I had done to myself. He made me put my name at the top of the list.

In making this list, and in taking action to correct the wrongs of the past, I stirred up memories of some things I had done and some things I hadn't done that I should've done as a responsible, productive member of society. It was a tough process to go through, just as taking my moral inventory had been a tough process.

As I started making this list and thinking about the people I'd harmed, the signs and the symptoms were all there. I identified where I was wrong. I wrote down ideas on how I could try to make it up to the people on the list.

When you commit to paper how badly you've hurt others, when you see it there, spelled out in front of you, it hurts a lot. And you can't use drugs anymore to medicate the pain you feel. This is one of the biggest steps you will take.

Have you harmed anyone in the course of your active addiction to this habit you want to be free of? Family, friends, your employer, your coworkers, your landlord, teachers, casual acquaintances, total strangers—think of anyone in your life you may have harmed because of your addiction. Don't forget to include yourself! Are you willing to make amends to the people on this list? Are you willing to make amends with yourself?

EXERCISE #8: MAKING AMENDS

Now it's your turn. Make a list of all the people who have been adversely affected by your active addiction (including yourself). Next to their names, write one word categorizing what the harm was—financial, moral, professional, familial, health, even human kindness in general. Next to that, write some suggestions for how you could attempt to correct that harm.

NAME	TYPE OF HARM	HOW CAN I CORRECT THE SITUATION?

NAME	TYPE OF HARM	HOW CAN I CORRECT THE SITUATION?

It's okay if you don't know right this moment how you're going to make amends. The important part of this step is seeing on paper what you did during active addiction that negatively impacted others, and who those people you harmed are. When you sit with this list awhile and process what you have written down, then you can start thinking about what you can do to make amends.

Taking action to fix things means disciplining yourself to commit to paper those things you've done to others.* We are not going to receive forgiveness from everyone we reach out to, but the point of this exercise is to admit to yourself what you've done and to actively try to fix your wrongdoings.

*Note: Because this process can be extremely painful, it's advised that you connect with your sponsor and do it with them.

The Principle of Forgiveness

- *Forgiveness*: to cease to feel resentment against (an offender); to pardon.
- *Forgiveness*: to give up resentment or claim to requital.

All of the principles we've covered so far—Honesty, Hope, Faith, Courage, Integrity, Willingness, Humility, and Discipline and Action—all build up to the principle of Forgiveness.

When we take the ninth step, the first person we have to ask forgiveness of is ourselves. If we can't forgive ourselves, we can't expect that anyone else will forgive us. If we can't forgive ourselves, we can't live.

I told you that my nana and granddaddy John kept me alive—literally—when I had given up. They gave me a place to stay, kept me off the street, gave me food and made sure I ate it. When I would come in, my nana would embrace me with excitement. She'd tell me she was happy to see me and happy that I was alive. "Sit down and get something to eat!" she'd tell me, and she'd make me something to eat. That was the kind of love I rarely got in my childhood, especially after I turned bad. But no matter what I had been up to, my nana and granddaddy John always made sure I knew they loved me.

Some of the things I did to them while I was under the influence of drugs were hurtful. I had to accept that I had done horrible things to these people who loved me. I had to realize that I was not responsible for my addiction, but that I was responsible for my recovery. Addiction was a sickness that had overtaken me. In my right mind, I never would have done some of the things I did—to my grandparents or anyone else. Understanding that truth allowed me to forgive myself.

My grandparents didn't live to see my recovery. More than twenty years ago, my nana developed kidney issues and fell into a coma for a few weeks. The doctors didn't think she was going to make it out of the coma and my granddaddy John was sure she was going to die. After going to visit her the night she fell into that coma and after hearing what the doctors said, he literally went home from the hospital and died that night. Our only rationale was that he could not bear the thought of being alive without her, that's how much he loved his wife. They shared over forty-five years of marriage. The was the same kind of love that kept me alive.

Nana did come out of the coma three days later, and she lived another four years. When my nana finally died, I was so devastated that I could not even go to her funeral. I refused to see her like that, lying in a casket, lifeless. I just couldn't do it.

While both of these wonderful people had passed away by the time I made it through a successful recovery program, I still had to fully complete the step of forgiveness, so I had to ask their forgiveness for the pain I brought to them.

I wrote them a letter apologizing for my behavior. I told them how grateful I was for everything they did for me, and how much I appreciated their love. One way for me to show them how grateful I was for all that they had done, even though they were no longer here, was to live my life in a way that would make them proud. In that letter, I also asked for their forgiveness.

I also needed to ask my daughters for forgiveness. I told you way back in the beginning of this book that what made me give my recovery another shot was my daughters. I did not want them growing up having to hear people say, "Your dad is a crackhead." That was one of the greatest motivating factors for me.

When I first tried to ask my eldest daughter, Raven, for forgiveness, she was in her early teens. At that point, I was not trying to be her daddy, but I wanted to have a line of communication with her and let her know I was a different person today—that I was a responsible, productive member of society, and that I wanted to be a part of her life.

She didn't accept my apology, and she didn't offer her forgiveness. I understood why, but it still hurt.

After that, I would call her, and she would talk to me, but if I asked her a question, she'd give me only one-word answers. We rarely had a real conversation. I started doing this my first year clean. Years later, it's still this way.

My mom and others have told me, "Well, you just got to keep trying."

What I realized when I talked to my sponsor was that the reason I kept trying was because I hadn't forgiven myself for not being there for her, and for all the broken promises I'd made to her. I was there in the beginning of her life, but then I made some wicked, bad decisions and I was a no-show for her toddler years and school years. I was trying to make good on those broken promises, but I couldn't.

I couldn't just pop up and say, "Daddy's here now." She wasn't having any of that.

I asked the Lord what to do. His response was that He doesn't force Himself on anybody and neither should I.

My sponsor told me to forgive myself for what I'd done. I'd caused her some harm, and he pointed out that it might be painful for her to talk to me. "If she's doing well, be happy for her. You continue to live the lifestyle that you live and allow her to have access to you. Make sure she has your number where she can reach you if she needs to, but if she chooses not to have a line of communication or a relationship with you, accept that. Forgive yourself and live your life."

I was a different person when I was in active addiction. I lived a foul lifestyle. Now I'm leading a clean and sober and moral life, but that doesn't mean someone else can forgive the damage that's been done. I've accepted the fact that if my daughters are better off without my presence, then I need to leave them alone. If my being a part of their lives causes them emotional pain and hurt and the bad memories are causing them more harm than good, then I need to move on.

When I met Paula, one of the most loving and caring women I have ever met and the future mother of my daughter Danielle, I had been clean for about a year. But I went back out, and I started using again. After Danielle was born, Paula took her back to Turks and Caicos to raise her around her family. I moved to Turks and Caicos for two years to be with them.

I thought I wouldn't use dope anymore because I was in a new place. Well, I got over there, and guess who was there when I got there? Me. I took me and my bad habits with me. I smoked dope and my relationship with Danielle and her mother went up in smoke. Literally.

I tried to develop a line of communication with Danielle over the years I've been clean. She and Raven have gotten together a few times. Raven even went to Danielle's high school graduation. Both of my girls have struggled to make sense of the broken relationship they have with me, so I was disconnected from both of my daughters for a while.

Danielle wouldn't answer when I called, so I left her alone and stopped calling. Her mother reached out to me on Facebook and told me to call again. I did. We started talking for a while but we stopped again. She says she forgave me, so I have to accept that and I have to let it go.

I practice forgiveness with my current wife. We all come with baggage, and I didn't understand some of her struggles when we were first married. There were some things that she did that weren't right, but I had to practice forgiveness. She asked for forgiveness, just like I had asked my daughters for forgiveness, and I knew that I had to grant it to her. The Bible says, we ought to forgive others if we expect God to forgive us.

Step 9:
We made direct amends to such people wherever possible,
except when to do so would injure them or others.

When we don't understand and practice forgiveness, we leave ourselves open to being ruled by our shortcomings. Without having forgiveness, if somebody harms me, my first instinct is to cause them harm back. With forgiveness, I cause no harm. I don't feel like I have to get back at anyone. I no longer feel like I have to inflict harm because I was harmed.

This transformation does not happen automatically. It takes practice. I didn't get to the point where I am today in my first year of recovery. We don't start off saying, "I'm going to turn the other cheek, no matter what." It's a process, and you have to develop the skills.

I asked Danielle for forgiveness for not being there for her, and after time, she granted it to me. I asked other people whom I had caused harm for forgiveness and many of them granted it to me. Not all. That's okay. Asking forgiveness is an act of kindness to myself as well. I get to release that negative energy. Just by asking for forgiveness, I free myself from the hurt, harm, and pain I've caused.

What is the worst thing you think will happen when you begin asking people for forgiveness? What is the worst thing that can happen if you never ask them for forgiveness? Which price are you willing to pay? If it's going to cause more harm, leave it alone. If it's going to open a wound that's already been healed, leave it alone.

EXERCISE #9: ASKING FORGIVENESS

Now you have your list. Now it's time to act on it. Take the list you made in the last exercise and add another column to it.

NAME	TYPE OF HARM	HOW CAN I CORRECT THE SITUATION?	WHEN CAN I CORRECT THE SITUATION?

NAME	TYPE OF HARM	HOW CAN I CORRECT THE SITUATION?	WHEN CAN I CORRECT THE SITUATION?

Adding "when" to the equation now makes forgiveness less of a concept and more of an action. Your response to "When?" could be "Right away" or "By their next birthday" or even "Never." The point is to have an actionable plan and a list of goals you can check off, rather than just a wish that someday you can make things right again. Remember that you're not guaranteed forgiveness just because you ask for it. But know that in the act of asking forgiveness, you perform an act of kindness for yourself.

Chapter Seven: Grow Up

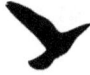

We now come to the last three steps and the principles that support us on our road to recovery. This section, "Grow Up," features the steps we need to take to ensure these principles of recovery becomes as firmly rooted in us as the bad habits of active addiction once were. Once you get through these steps and start living these principles, you will be firmly on your way to living a life free from active addiction and fully freeing yourself from yourself.

The Principle of Acceptance
- *Accept:* to receive (something offered) willingly; to be able or designed to take or hold (something applied or added).
- *Accept:* to give admittance or approval to.
- *Accept:* to endure without protest or reaction; to regard as proper, normal, or inevitable; to recognize as true; to believe.
- *Accept:* to make a favorable response to; to agree to undertake (a responsibility).

Do you know how hunters catch monkeys? They put a coconut in a trap. The monkey will reach in there and grab the coconut, and with his fist around the coconut, he can't get his arm out. If he just lets go of the coconut, he can free himself from the trap and get his arm through the hole again. He can break free before he's captured if he just lets go. But many monkeys won't let go of the coconut, so they get captured.

That's what an addiction does to people—it captures them through their unwillingness to let go. It captured me. It caused me to lose everything, to the point where I almost lost me. By the time I got to my twelfth rehab, I was ready to lose me. I didn't know how to live, and I didn't know how to free myself from myself.

The 12-step program says acceptance is the antidote to all our problems. Acceptance is big in recovering from addiction. Acceptance allows us to be imperfect—to be human. Acceptance allows us to understand that other people are human. When we know that we have done our best, and we have given our all, we can leave the rest up to our Higher Power. To some, that's God. To me, that's G.O.D.—Good Orderly Direction, applying the system of unchangeable principles I use to guide me.

When I don't accept people for who they are, that means I'm trying to control them. When I place unrealistic expectations on others in an attempt to control them, they usually don't meet my expectations. And guess what happens next? I breed resentments against this person. Then I have to bear the burden of these resentments, anger directed inward. If I could accept this person for who they are, I would not have to live with this resentment.

Just because I accept someone for who they are doesn't mean I can't communicate my displeasure with their behavior. I can tell someone, "Hey, you wronged me," or "I don't agree with that," and I can still accept who they are. When I accept another person for who they are, I take away the possibility that I will feel anger or resentment, which then may turn into a negative action or a shortcoming for me.

I can show others exactly how to change their situation and condition, but not if they don't want to change, and I have to accept the fact that another person may not want to change. I have to accept that they choose to live the lifestyle they live, and that relieves the pressure on me.

Step 10:
We continued to take personal inventory and
when we were wrong promptly admitted it.

Like forgiveness, practicing acceptance meant I also needed to accept myself. This step challenged me to accept the mistakes I made in life. To be clear, we don't have to be okay with these mistakes. But we need to acknowledge that they happened and accept that they happened. We can't go back and change the past. We'll only frustrate ourselves if we try, and that frustration may trigger another shortcoming.

Instead, we can look honestly at the present moment and work with what we have. I could accept that I had lost jobs. I could accept what I had done to my nana and my granddaddy John. I could accept that I had not lived my life to my potential. By accepting myself and my shortcomings, I was able to learn how to accept other people's mistakes when they fell short. How could I get mad with someone for being who they were?

For so many years, I didn't accept the fact that I was an addict. Had I accepted my reality as an addict, I could have saved myself a lot of years of active addiction, and lots of money and heartache for my friends and family.

Even in rehab, I could not accept that I was an addict the first eleven times. I told myself I took too many drugs, but I wasn't an addict. I could not accept that truth. When it was time to introduce myself in a Narcotics Anonymous meeting, I'd say, "My name is Tim and I'm in recovery." I never said, "My name is Tim, and I'm an addict." I never accepted that I was an addict; therefore, my recovery never worked.

The first step is to admit that we are addicts. Only through admitting there's a problem will we ever arrive at acceptance.

To avoid going back to denying reality, I do a personal moral inventory every day, like the one I took you through earlier. I check my thoughts. I check the words that I speak. I check my motives. I look at the part that I play in any given situation. I look at how my character defect of pride—maybe I got defensive with my boss over something—became a shortcoming the minute I opened my mouth. I look at what I did, and I accept that I was wrong. I think about how I could have handled the situation differently, and how I will handle a similar situation differently in the future.

I will say this again and again: these steps are ongoing. They are not one and done. We practice these principles in all of our affairs and on a daily basis. That's how we maintain sobriety. These principles protect us from ourselves.

In Step 4, we did a searching and fearless moral inventory, which means that we wrote everything down—things that we would have taken to our grave. The program teaches us that if we don't reveal or admit our darkest, deepest secrets to ourselves, that unacknowledged pain can resurface or trigger at unexpected moments, causing us to want to get high again. Writing things down for ourselves doesn't mean we broadcast everything, but we face what we've done, and we give ourselves a plan to deal with the damage.

It's therapeutic to release pain and hurt with another person. Have you ever heard the term "stuffing feelings"? When we stuff feelings, we're not accepting what we're feeling. We don't know how to deal with these feelings, so we stuff them back down into ourselves. Have you ever heard about somebody who has been raped, and they just block it out and don't remember it? Stuffing feelings can become a habit, but after a while, it all comes back up. When that happens, it can be so much more of a load to bear that the person can't handle it. Many times, it can result in that person doing something destructive—like abusing drugs and alcohol.

Remember how Dr. Myles Monroe talked about us having a conscious and a subconscious mind? Our subconscious is what monitors our heart rate, breathing, and other things so we don't even have to think about it. It's all automatic. The conscious mind is like a computer, processing information that comes in. When we hear the same thing over and over again, it is downloaded from our conscious mind into our subconscious mind—which is sometimes referred to as our heart because it keeps running automatically to keep us alive. Now it becomes part of our heart, and once it gets there, it's like hell trying to get it out of there. It's not impossible, though. You just have to accept that it got in there and then you have to do the work to shake it out of there.

Many people won't free themselves from themselves because it takes a lot of work to download and process all the principles and effectively change what's in our hearts. It requires daily maintenance. We have to be proactive with it, like going to the doctor for a physical or taking our car in for a tune-up. We have to keep it in check, like watching our diet.

We've been talking a lot about how the steps work and why they are important, but really, practicing the principles means setting goals to plan for a better life—a higher quality of life, and one we can achieve if we do the work. In order to do that, we must accept that we have to do the work.

Are you ready to accept the truth that you have a problem that you can fix if you do the work? Are you willing to accept these principles into your life and download and process them into your soul to become a better person?

Completing this program is like performing surgery on yourself, and it has to be done delicately. But you can do it, and you can become a better person for it. Accept, do your maintenance, and heal.

EXERCISE #10: SWOT ANALYSIS

In business, there's a system companies use called a SWOT analysis that helps keep things running smoothly. SWOT stands for Strengths, Weaknesses, Opportunities, Threats.

To avoid going back to denying reality, I constantly do a personal inventory, or what my sponsor calls a self-analysis. I check my actions. I check my thoughts. I check the words that I speak. I do a SWOT analysis to keep myself in check. At the end of the day, I ask myself, "Who did you hurt today?" and "Who did you help today?" Now it's your turn.

At the end of the day, add your actions to each of these columns.

- If you did something good, list that under Strengths.
- If you did something you're not so proud of, that goes under Weaknesses.
- If you saw a way you could make a positive change, that goes under Opportunities.
- And if something came into your life that may have triggered a shortcoming, list that under Threats.

STRENGTHS	WEAKNESSES	OPPORTUNITIES	THREATS

STRENGTHS	WEAKNESSES	OPPORTUNITIES	THREATS

When you look at this inventory every day, you'll start to see patterns emerge. These patterns will show you what areas you're strongest in, and what areas you're less strong in. When you see all this written out on paper, you'll be better able to accept who you've been, who you are, and who you are becoming.

The Principle of Knowledge and Awareness

- *Knowledge:* the fact or condition of knowing something with familiarity gained through experience or association.
- *Knowledge:* acquaintance with or understanding of a science, art, or technique; the fact or condition of being aware of something; the range of one's information or understanding; the circumstance or condition of apprehending truth or fact through reasoning; cognition; the fact or condition of having information or of being learned.
- *Knowledge:* the sum of what is known; the body of truth, information, and principles acquired by humankind.
- *Awareness:* realization, perception, or knowledge.

Knowledge and Awareness are important; they help us discover how to become better people. We have to look for the information that helps us to improve; we have to be aware that we are processing the right information in the right way, and doing the work to make us better people.

Spirituality and religion have different answers for the kind of work we have to do. Religion says we need to join a church. Churches have a doctrinal statement on what they believe, and it basically has to do with the "guy in the sky." If we question what they believe, if we don't accept their idea of what God means to them, you will probably be asked to leave.

Spirituality is the basis of the 12-step program. It doesn't operate like religion. Spirituality means we accept a Higher Power—that something greater than ourselves can guide you—but that Higher Power does not have to be the same God as in religion. I've met people whose Higher Power was a doorknob. Why? Because a doorknob opens doors for them. For some people, the Higher Power is the group. Your higher power will be something that guides, directs, and helps you—something bigger than yourself that you can put your trust in, because you have evidence that it leads to healthy thoughts and healthy crops and keeps the weeds away.

We have knowledge of a Higher Power, and we are aware that because we attribute strength to that Higher Power, we have an awareness that this power can guide us, no matter what we choose for it to be.

Think of it this way. Imagine a ninety-pound police officer standing in the road and stopping a hundred cars. This guy is ninety pounds soaking wet, but in this traffic jam, he is the higher power. The drivers accept his presence as a greater power, and they do what he tells them to do because of the authority in the badge he wears. He can't physically stop them, but because the drivers are aware of this authority, having to do with his badge, they know and understand that they need to stop because he is guiding them to do so.

Step 11 talks about God as we now understand what God wants for us:

Step 11:

We sought through prayer and meditation to improve our conscious contact with God as we understood Him, praying only for knowledge of His will for us and the power to carry that out.

When we communicate with God *as we understand Him*, we don't pray for God to change things. Prayer changes *you*, it doesn't change the things around you. We pray to establish our relationship and for understanding of what our Higher Power wants for us. We don't pray for cars, for money, or for help getting out of sticky situations. That's not what prayer is for as we understand it.

Prayer is for communicating our concerns to a power greater than ourselves. In NA, prayer is reaching out and asking our Higher Power for help. Prayer is the knowing that I need something.

Meditation is listening for the answer. Meditation is the awareness that I will get the instructions to get what I need.

When I pray, I ask my Higher Power to help me understand my gift, my purpose for being on this planet, and I ask for the knowledge, wisdom, and understanding to carry out that purpose.

Meditation helps me understand the true nature of my gifts and how to use them to help others. When I meditate, I also often receive guidance on how to sow the seed of my gifts so thick in my words, thoughts, and actions, that the weed seeds have no room to take root and prevent me from prospering.

Once I got clean and I got out of that twelfth treatment center, I watched Joyce Meyers at 5:30 and Creflo Dollar preach on TV at 6:00

every morning with notebook and paper. They both helped me gain a deeper understanding of many biblical stories, and that understanding helped me uncover the spiritual principles embedded in those parables. There were things they preached that I didn't understand and that I still question, but as they tell us in the program, "If it don't apply, let it fly." Think of it this way: If you have this big pretty apple with one small brown spot on it, you don't throw the whole apple away. You cut the brown spot out, and you enjoy the apple. You can do the same with knowledge. Keep the advice that is helpful to you and discard the rest.

I built my knowledge. I started studying the Bible and taking notes and learning solid principles to live by. I eventually came to the point that it did not matter to me whether the stories really happened. I needed to understand the moral principles behind the stories so I could learn how to make better decisions and stop self-medicating. The story of Moses splitting the Red Sea wasn't going to help me stop smoking crack. Instead, I focused on principles like seed, time, and harvest, I thought about every seed producing after its own kind, and I meditated on the laws that govern life. The Bible became a manual for me.

"In the beginning was the Word, and the Word was with God, and the Word was God" (1 John 1:1). And so this word, this manual, this knowledge, became my Higher Power. With the Bible, I could hold God in my hand and sow God into my heart.

I was never really taught how to pray or have a conscious contact with God in my earlier years of attending church. This contact with God is a newer addition to my life. Now, when I go walking, I feel the energy of the universe. I am aware of everything around me. I take it all in, and I understand that everything is designed to be in harmony. We're never going to see a tree limb fighting another tree limb—they live in harmony together, wanting the best for each other.

As I continue to be in conscious contact with God, I see the manifestations of my Creator everywhere in nature. I am aware that everything in nature is a manifestation of the same Creator who created me. The principle of seed, time, and harvest, and the lawn analogy—they are all nature-based. They are all principles of the natural world that God set in motion and that will never change. They will be the same today, yesterday, and forevermore.

Through my knowledge and awareness of this conscious contact with what I understand as God, I've come to feel that God lives inside of me. I no longer pray outward; I pray inward. I don't buy the "Jesus is gonna fix it" methodology. No, God won't fix it, but God will give me instructions. God's spirit lives inside of me and has given me the ability to create the change that I need to create in my life. Through this manual, I have God's instructions and help. However, it's my responsibility to do the hard work of changing. That's my part.

To discover my gift and God's purpose for me, I had to ask myself some important questions, which I learned from Dr. Myles Munroe:

- Who am I? (Identity)
- Why am I here? (Purpose)
- What can I do that speaks to my purpose? (Potential)

When I discover my gift, it simultaneously brings purpose to my life. I like to talk. My gift of speaking is my gift. When I ask and answer these questions asked by Dr. Myles Munroe, I understand God's purpose for me.

When I left my final rehab center, I created a new habit of learning about God through TV ministries and reading the Bible to help me gain the knowledge and awareness I needed to continue working toward my freedom. By focusing my prayer on learning His will for me and by asking for the power to carry it out, I started becoming aware of the harmony in nature and began to make sense of my connection to it.

What do you have access to around you to help you gain the knowledge and awareness you'll need to maintain your freedom? Are you ready to seek out a connection that can help you discover your place in this world? What is stopping you from praying right now to ask for knowledge of God's will for your life and the power to carry it out?

EXERCISE #11: DISCOVERING YOUR PURPOSE

We developed a list of questions for the Free Yourself From Yourself program that can help you discover your gift and get on your path to becoming the person you are meant to be, which I will share here with you. Answer these questions in the space provided:

What is your deepest desire?

_____

_____

_____

What's your wish for humanity?

_____

_____

_____

What's your deepest passion?

_____

_____

_____

What do you think about when you're alone?

_____

_____

What do you wish you could change in your community?

_____

_____

_____

What would you do if you had unlimited resources?

_____

_____

_____

What comes naturally for you?

_____

_____

_____

What would you do for no pay?

_____

_____

_____

The answers you provide to these questions will bring you closer to knowing what your gift is and set you on a path toward living it.

The Principle of Service and Gratitude

- *Service*: the occupation or function of serving.
- *Service*: the work performed by one that serves; help, use, benefit; contribution to the welfare of others.
- *Service*: the act of serving; a helpful act; useful labor that does not produce a tangible commodity.
- *Gratitude:* appreciation of benefits received; an expression of gratefulness.

A big part of why I show up to meetings is for the newcomers to see that the program works. I'm not beyond the 12-step program, because I'll always live this lifestyle. But a responsibility I have as a result of my success is to carry this message to people who are still caught up in the grips of active addiction and struggling to come out of it.

The act of attending these meetings is both service and gratitude. I have gratitude for being able to finally come to the other side of active addiction. I am thankful every day that I found the path to bring me to the lifestyle I enjoy today.

Service comes into play in the service I provide to others by being at these meetings. Remember we talked earlier in our discussion of the principle of hope and how hearing the success stories of others had the ability to create a hope shot for those still struggling to overcome active addiction? When I attend NA meetings, and I share my story, it is an act of service to others who rely on these hope shots to keep going.

In the 12-step program, the steps are for individuals, and the 12 traditions are for our groups. The 12 traditions are guides for our service work, and they are recited at the beginning of every meeting. Reciting these traditions is non-negotiable because it really does help grow the grass seed nice and thick. I won't list all of the traditions here, but I would like to call attention to tradition five, which is one of the best examples of the principles of service and gratitude: "Each group has but one primary purpose—to carry the message to the addict who still suffers." Because we have strength in our gratitude to not be using and living the active addiction lifestyle, we have the purpose to serve others who are still struggling. We do this by sharing our stories with them.

Step 12:

Having had a spiritual awakening as a result of these steps, we tried to carry this message to addicts, and to practice these principles in all our affairs.

Five years into my new clean life, I had gone from sleeping on the floor in a homeless shelter to living in a 2,400-square-foot home—a really nice home, in a nice neighborhood. And this is me, the same person who once crawled around on the floor looking for crack rocks. I'm married. I have a career. I'm a responsible, productive member of society.

I asked God, "What do I do now? I'm living clean. I've got a different lifestyle. I've figured out how to live and not get high. And I've seen some different results in my life. But what do I do now?"

In other words, "I am grateful for this clean and sober lifestyle. Now how can I serve others to live and show that gratitude?"

This time, I asked myself a question: "What gifts did my Creator give me?"

In the last step, I had already started thinking about my purpose, and this question drove me to think about it even more. I had always loved to talk and now I really had something positive to talk about. Back in my elementary school years, I was often punished by my teachers, being sent in front of the classroom, to put my nose in a circle drawn on the chalkboard for talking in class. I was always talking and making my classmates laugh.

So, my gift is talking and sharing. That's what I came up with as my purpose—speaking to inspire others. I even developed a brand name, TalkManTalk, which I modeled after Michael Jordon's brand Jumpman.

I also realized that the principles I learned could be helpful to my family members, friends, and coworkers. Even if they don't use dope, they could still benefit from this program. I decided I was going to serve by helping others understand these principles—a living, breathing example of how life can drastically improve when any human begins to accept change based on these principles.

This book and this program are my ways of carrying this message to the world. This book and my program are what I do. *Free Yourself From Yourself* is just a part of the service work I provide to other recovering addicts and to the world. My gift is being able to share what I've learned in order to help others. That's what I do, and I'm good at it. It's my gift. I am extremely grateful to have discovered one of my most precious gifts, and I celebrate that gratitude by sharing it.

I share my spirituality and strength and hope with other addicts, as many of us on this side of recovery do. We do service work, but it's not just about helping others to start living a life of freedom from active addiction. It's for us to keep remembering where we came from, and to keep walking away from that and toward being better people.

Taking time to share with others is a two-way street. There's an important phrase: "We keep what we have by giving it away." When I tell others my stories, or when I share these principles, not only does the other person hear and benefit from my words, but I hear and benefit from them as well. They serve as a reminder of where I've been and where I want to go. I'm reminded that I never want to be stuck in that vicious cycle of pain again. In other words, I'm constantly sowing the grass seed thick. I continue to sow the right seeds in my ear, which are then planted deep down in my soul. When I get up in the morning and I look in the mirror, I remember that user who would stare in the mirror with contempt for what they saw—that person who would grab the Listerine out of the medicine cabinet behind the mirror and try to drink away the pain and disgust they felt coming face-to-face with their own reflection.

Today, I have a job, a wife, a home. I have a career as a motivational speaker and life coach. I help others start on the pathway toward healing, so they can like what they see when they look in the mirror. I have the deepest sense of gratitude for these spiritual principles, which helped me like, and then love, the person I see in the mirror.

Service work gives us the opportunity to connect to people who are like us. We no longer live selfishly. Service means using our gifts to help others. It is the reason our gifts were given to us in the first place.

Connecting to others and seeing how far we've come helps us feel gratitude. Gratitude is the attitude that keeps us thriving and strong. Service reminds us where we've come from and gratitude grounds us in where we're headed.

When we focus on the things we're grateful for, we are overseeding our lawns with the right seeds, which yield good thoughts, which lead to good deeds, which then develop into healthy habits and behaviors. At the same time, we are choking out the negative thoughts like jealousy, resentment, and fear. In short, gratitude is health food for our souls.

This book and the Free Yourself From Yourself program are my ways of carrying this message to the world. This is my service work, and I'm grateful to share my work with you.

What's yours?

EXERCISE #12: PRACTICING GRATITUDE

No matter how bad things get, as long as you can find something to be grateful for, you're going to be okay. You can practice gratitude for something as small as the milk in your refrigerator not being past its expiration date. You can practice gratitude for something that you may take for granted, like that you have a clean shirt on your back. You can practice gratitude for something enormous, like getting a new job or reaching a sobriety milestone. There is nothing too big or too small to be grateful for.

This last exercise in the book is simple. I want you to write on the list five things you are grateful for, and I want you to do this every night before you go to sleep.

1. _____

_____

2. _____

_____

3._____

_____

4. _____

_____

5. _____

_____

The more gratitude you can feel, the better you can heal.

CLOSING THOUGHTS

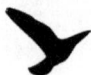

Now that you've discovered the principles that are the foundation of the 12-step program to recovering from addiction, it's up to you to put them into practice. I've outlined what they are, and shared examples of where I was before I opened myself to these guiding principles. I've also challenged you to get started working on them.

Getting to recovery is not going to happen in the pages of a quick (and, I hope, entertaining) book. The book is designed to give you an introduction to what living a clean and sober lifestyle takes, but it doesn't stop when you close this book and put it down. Recovery is a process you will be living every day now, and for the rest of your life. Your commitment to recovery is one of the biggest commitments you will ever make.

The Free Yourself From Yourself program provides ongoing support for you as you navigate your way through this important, at times difficult, but ultimately rewarding process. If you're ready to take your recovery seriously, reach out today and I will be your coach to winning your life back from active addiction once and for all: freeyourselffromyourself.com.

WE DO RECOVER!
Let's start today.

ADDITIONAL INFORMATION

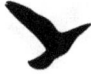

For information regarding booking Timothy as a recovery coach or motivational speaker, please email info@talkmantalk.com.

To learn more about TalkManTalk Publishing and all its affiliated programs, please visit talkmantalk.com.

For more information about the author or upcoming FYFY events, please visit freeyourselffromyourself.com.

MY NANA

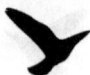

My grandmother was a dear sweet lady
Showing me honest and sincere love
From the time I was a baby
She had a heart as pure as gold
One of those saints from old
She sang, she preached, and would even shout
She praised God; the very thing Jesus was about
It was no secret that I was her favorite
And this I won't deny, however
She loved everyone unconditionally
An act many so-called saints should try
Family members told her, "Put Timothy out and let him go"
But she was a follower of Jesus Christ and when I showed up
She said, "Come on in and close the door"
God gave her the tools to defeat Satan and win
Even though she wasn't perfect
She was still human; still subject to sin
She wore fine clothes, how she loved to dress
And was a master in the kitchen
Her fried chicken was the best
She lived for Jesus, to Him her life she gave
Her body will go in the dirt, but her spirit won't be in that grave
Her life on this earth has finally come to an end
And yes, I will miss her
She was not only my grandmother, she was my friend

I must say goodbye for now
But this is not the end
God has answered her prayer and saved me
I will see her again

www.ingramcontent.com/pod-product-compliance
Lightning Source LLC
Chambersburg PA
CBHW071954070426
42453CB00008BA/756